CONTENTS

Chapter 3: The Baby's Development

Chapter 4: The Many Faces of the Expectant Father

Chapter 5: The Body of the Pregnant Woman

Chapter 6: The Mind of the Pregnant Woman

Chapter 7: Spoiling Your Pregnant Partner

Helping Her Feel as Good as She Feels Big **221**

Chapter 8: Pregnant Sex

Having It, Not Having It,

Fantasizing about Having It **245**

Chapter 9: Shopping for Baby

Something So Little Needs So Much **261**

Chapter 10: Passing the Time

Things to Do During the Second

and Third Trimesters **287**

Chapter 11: Labor and Delivery Prep Time

Things to Help Prepare You

for Labor and Delivery **323**

Chapter 12: The Birth Day

From Your Door to Delivery Room
and Back Again **363**

Chapter 13: After the Baby Is Born

The Fourth Trimester Begins **415**

THANK YOU FOR HELPING ME GIVE BIRTH...

I'd like to thank Stephanie, my pregnant wife/best friend/inspiration/partner/editor/love of my life. Thank you for letting me test my theories and hypotheses on you during all three of your pregnancies. You are the most beautiful pregnant woman in the world. In fact, from behind, you never looked pregnant. I'd like to thank my daughter, Eva Kaye, and sons Harrison and Asher. Thank you for being so well-behaved, warm-hearted, and kind in the womb (and outside). You are the greatest gift in the world and it's a privilege to be your daddy. Mommy and I love you so much. (P.S. If we mess up, let us know and we'll make things better or get you the very best therapy available.) Thank you to my mom (Shirlee) and dad (Eugene) for creating me and to my mom for giving birth to me. In fact, I'd like to take this opportunity to formally apologize to you, Mom. Sorry I was two weeks overdue and that I had to be delivered via a surprise C-section. I don't know what I was thinking—if I could do it all over again I'd have popped out at seven and a half pounds and saved you the scar. Who knows, I might even have a younger sibling had it been easier. Please accept my apology. I love you. And thank you, Dad, for being the best father in the world. While you didn't get a chance to cut the cord because you weren't invited into the delivery room (I'll find you some kind of cord to cut later if you want), I love you as much as a son can love his dad. I'd like to thank my in-laws Fran and Marvin. I believe that if you could have given birth to me, you would have done it, but instead, you gave birth to my wife—and that's more than enough for me. Your constant love, support, and encouragement are a gift. Thank you to my big brothers, Vic and Michael, and older sister-in-law Irene—your wisdom, advice, guidance, help, love, hand-me downs, and breast pump were so deeply appreciated (clarification—the breast pump was from Irene). Thank you to my younger brother-in-law Dan and sister-in-law Rozi. I hope, as your (BBIL) big-brother-in-law, I can teach you the ways of the world. Thanks for all the love and always being there for us. Thank you to my nieces Phoebe, Rae, and Hannah and my nephews Henry and Ethan. You have been the cutest and best practice babies for Steph and me. I love being your uncle. A heartfelt thank-you goes out to friends, family, and all the random contributors I accosted while researching this book. Thank you for opening up your lives and sharing your most personal, emotional, embarrassing, and deeply honest stories as part of this book. Your experiences are what make this project so compelling. Thank you to all the doctors, nurses, and caregivers who helped us through pregnancy, labor, and delivery and the pregnancy, labor, and delivery of this book. My deepest gratitude goes out to my longtime editorial obstetrician, Peter Lynch, and my new editorial obstetrics team of Stephanie Bowen and Jenna Skwarek. You are all gifted handlers of thoughts, ideas, and words—thank you for helping me push and deliver this book from my womb (again, no editing). Thanks to Todd Stocke (director of editorial obstetrics), and the editorial, sales, publicity, and support teams at Sourcebooks. A heartfelt thank-you goes out to Dominique Raccah, chief editorial obstetrician (Sourcebooks's publisher). Your passion, commitment, and encouragement are an inspiration. A thank-you goes out to my agent/midwife, Eliot Ephraim. You continue to be right there by my side throughout the personal and professional journey. Thank you to Glenn Mott and the entire team at King Features Syndicate, the newspaper editors who have supported my "Help Me, Harlan!" syndicated advice column over the years, the readers of "Help Me, Harlan!," the students and professionals who have invited me to share my passion on college campuses over the years, the Indiana University School of Journalism, the *Indiana Daily Student*, and the late Dr. Dave Adams (still can't believe you're gone—I miss you).

Finally, thank you to the readers of this book. It's a privilege to have the opportunity to share this experience and time with you. I look forward to what I hope will be the beginning of a long relationship with you as you experience the most amazing, profound, surreal, and awesome adventure of your life.

Thank you!
Harlan Cohen

THE CONCEPTION

HOW IT HAPPENED...

It might have happened on your honeymoon, on vacation, on a first date, in an elevator, on an escalator, on the bathroom floor, on the kitchen counter, in the bedroom, after senior prom, at a friend's wedding, at your own wedding, in a doctor's office, at a fertility clinic, with the help of a surrogate, or through an adoption agency. It might have happened on purpose, by accident, or by chance. It could have been a broken condom, a missed pill, a romantic evening, a one-night stand, a fluke, or a well-orchestrated plan involving ovulation kits and basal thermometers. You might have been trying for minutes, days, weeks, months, or years. You might be single. You might be married. You might be separated. You might be in love, in lust, in like, or neither. The news might be shocking, scary, exciting, overwhelming, or not *real* considering not much has changed (assuming you're in the first trimester). How it happened, when it happened, where it happened, or why it happened is all in the past. All that matters is that it's happened. What you will encounter next is *the most* exhilarating, emotional, intense, intimidating, and awesome experience of your entire life.

Congratulations!

The following pages will offer a rarely seen look into the expectant father experience. It's everything a dad-to-be can expect to see, hear, feel, touch, taste, and smell (see Tip #36). It's everything that the partner of a dad-to-be needs to know to understand what he's thinking, what he's doing, and what he's not doing.

Never before in the history of men and women have expectant fathers been so involved in the pregnancy process. From conception to delivery, men are attending appointments, holding legs, helping her push, positioning mirrors, cutting cords, changing diapers, taking care of our partners, comforting and feeding baby, and doing it all. While women expect us to be more involved and helpful than ever before, there's so little information to help us know what to do and how to do it. While women have hundreds of years of oral and written history handed down from generation to generation, today's expectant fathers are the first generation living in this unprecedented time in history. Other than our friends telling us over and over again, "You have no idea how life will change, man," we have little more to go on.

As a three-time expectant father, I know what it's like

to be there. I also know what it's like to wish you had known something ahead of time. That's what this book is all about—everything you need to know that you didn't know you needed to know. Some of it is obvious, some of it is new, but all of it is something you'll want to know.

Dad's Expecting Too is a living piece of work. The second edition includes new tips, stories, facts, and stats based on reader feedback. If you have a resource that's helped you, send it my way. If you have a story, advice, or tip—send it over. Email me at Harlan@helpmeharlan.com or Harlan @DadsExpectingToo.com. You can also submit your stories and tips via www.DadsExpectingToo.com. Also, please check out the Dad's Expecting Too Facebook page.

Again, thank you for picking up this book. I look forward to sharing this experience with you. Enjoy the adventure…it's a wild ride.

Thank you!
Harlan Cohen

WELCOME, EXPECTANT FATHERS

As a three-time expectant father, I know the last thing most men want to do is read a book for expectant fathers. I get it. I'm right there with you. That's why I wrote this thing. This book will not suck. You can read it from cover to cover, skip around, or keep it next to your bed to give the appearance you're reading.

If you were reading this book forty years ago, it would be smaller and simpler. Get her pregnant, go to work, have a kid, smoke a cigar. But in the past forty years, things have dramatically changed. Men are now expected to get her pregnant, go to doctors' appointments, register with her, listen, learn, and be as close to the action as possible before, during, and after delivery. We see it, hear it, feel it, touch it, and even smell it (not sure what smells).

From your first doctor's visit to holding her leg during delivery to catching a glimpse of her BV (birthing vagina) to holding your newborn fresh from the womb, we are pregnancy pioneers. As a result, women expect us to know more and do more. The problem is most of us have never done this before. We are treading in uncharted amniotic waters. We are the first generation of men expected to play this major of a role. And when you haven't done it before, and not a lot of people can guide you, it's hard to know what to say or what to do.

Dad's Expecting Too is about helping you to know what to expect so you can get comfortable with the uncomfortable. When you know what's coming, instead of elevating stress and being a nervous hysteric, you can relax and alleviate it. While all the situations in this book might not play out for you, many of them will. Simply knowing what's coming your way (even if you can't change it) will help you navigate the coming months with calmness and clarity.

As you page through this book, share information with your pregnant partner. Use it as an ongoing resource. For example, when attempting to have sex with your pregnant partner, flip to Tip #57 and bounce the seduction techniques off her. If it's too hard to hold the page in place while experimenting, use an iPad, Kindle, or e-reader. If she starts freaking out and getting scared about having a baby, Tip #47 will remind you to remind her that being scared is normal. You can even read her stories and quotes from other parents. If you feel like she's struggling emotionally, check out the depression Tip #49 and look for warning signs.

One more thing worth mentioning: I've included some pictures in this book (see Chapter 3). We are visual. Check out the week-by-week changes happening with your new baby and stay involved. While she has forty weeks to feel pregnant, we have to work to find ways to stay connected and engaged. I hope the images and information help.

As I mentioned in the intro, this is the second edition of what will be many more editions. If something bothers you, let me know. If there is a resource that's helped you, send it my way. If you don't appreciate my humor, suggest a better joke. If you have a story, advice, or tip—send it over. You can email me at Harlan@helpmeharlan.com or Harlan @DadsExpectingToo.com. You can also submit stories and tips via www.DadsExpectingToo.com. And when you're on Facebook, please check out the Dad's Expecting Too Facebook group.

Thank you!
Harlan

WELCOME, EXPECTANT MOTHERS

First, thank you for not making us give birth. That would be awful. I don't even know how the baby could come out (I can imagine). I'm still completely blown away by what you endure while going through this entire process. From start to birth, the female body is awesome. Creating life, carrying it for almost ten months, and then having to get it out of your body is something I can't even imagine. You are a hero.

While you're going through the most dramatic physical and emotional changes of your life, we are supposed to be there for you. We are supposed to say and do all the right things. We are supposed to take care of you and ourselves and remain cool the whole time. Let me tell you a secret—we are dealing with our own changes. I know you don't care, but we aren't cool. We want to be supportive, and we want to be helpful (at least most of us), but it's hard to know what to do or how to do it. It's our first time too.

While there are countless books for women dealing with pregnancy, there isn't one that focuses on the role of men and what women wish their partners would say or do to help make this experience more comfortable both physically and emotionally. That's what this book is about. It's what men are thinking and feeling. It's what their pregnant partners are thinking and feeling. It's what you need to know to better understand your man.

While interviewing women for this project, I'd ask them what their partners did right, did wrong, and could do better. Not only can you read the answers that other women have shared, the information should give you a little bit of insight into what your partner is feeling and how to help him better understand what you're going through.

As I've mentioned earlier, this is the second edition of many editions to follow. I'm sure there are many more issues, stories, and tips that should be included to help men get it right the first time. Please share your expert advice. If there are topics, tips, and suggestions you'd like to see in future editions, let me know. If there are things you'd like me to get rid of in future editions, let me know. You can email me at Harlan@helpmeharlan.com. You can also submit stories and tips via www.DadsExpectingToo.com and contribute to the expectant forums online at www.DadsExpectingToo.com. And if you're on Facebook, please check out the Dad's Expecting Too Facebook group.

Thank you!
Harlan

WELCOME, HEALTHCARE PROFESSIONALS

First, thank you for the work you do. With so many different personality types walking in and out of your offices and everyone's emotions running high (not to mention the premiums for insurance running high), it must be as thrilling as it is exhausting to do what you do on a daily basis. Your expertise and support is a gift.

As an expectant father who attended every prenatal appointment and talked to hundreds of parents who went through the same process, I have a much deeper appreciation of what it means to receive care when going through this experience. I hope this book can become an invaluable resource to help expectant men and women get comfortable with a naturally uncomfortable experience. I hope it will encourage them to ask questions freely, share their concerns with you, and feel more connected to their caregivers.

I did my very best to provide a balanced point of view. I made a concerted effort to avoid advocating one practice over another. I advocate patient education so that each individual can make an informed decision that's aligned with their values. I know this experience is a deeply personal and emotional one for patients and caregivers. If you come across something in this book that can be improved or better balanced, let me know. Likewise, if you love something, please let me know.

As I mentioned earlier, I like to think of this book as a living, breathing work (but you will not find a pulse using your Doppler). Please share any feedback you can offer. I would be thrilled to consider including your stories and tips (always anonymous) in future editions. Please email me at Harlan@helpmeharlan.com or via Harlan @DadsExpectingToo.com. You can also submit stories and tips via www.DadsExpectingToo.com and check out the weekly dad-to-be tracker. And when you're on Facebook, please check out the Dad's Expecting Too page.

Thank you!
Harlan

HOW THIS BOOK WAS PUT TOGETHER

As a syndicated advice columnist for the past eighteen years, people have been sharing their deepest secrets with me for my entire adult life. My favorite part of my advice column is sharing stories from people who have been there and lived it. It's the people who are living it or have recently lived it who are some of the most credible experts.

This book captures the voices of these experts—it's people who have lived it or have recently lived it sharing their tips, stories, and insight. As you go through your experience, I hope you will share your stories and insight as it unfolds. My goal is to provide the most complete look at the expectant father experience.

HOW THIS BOOK WAS RESEARCHED

- **I got someone pregnant**. Actually, we kind of planned it, so it worked out well. She was receptive to the idea. She had never been pregnant, and I had never gotten a woman pregnant, so it was all a new experience. My experience is central to this, but I'm just one of the guys who has been there and done it.

- **I got someone pregnant again.** Again, we kind of planned it so it made the process easier. Going through the experience for another time while writing this book was surreal. Having a little distance from the first experience and seeing how it unfolded the second time around helped to provide some clarity and put things in perspective.

- **I got someone pregnant one more time.** Yes, it was my wife again. Surprisingly, the third time has been the most uncomfortable. I thought I'd be cool with this process, but it's still unsettling. Writing and researching the second edition of this book calmed my nerves but stirred new concerns.

- **I interviewed expectant and new dads.** Over the life of this project, I've talked to hundreds of expectant dads. I posted requests online, spoke to people over the phone, and talked to people face-to-face. I asked them to share their tips and the stories behind the tips. Tips are suggestions lacking context—the stories behind the tip are where the real wisdom can be gleaned.

- **I interviewed expectant and new moms.** This was tricky. I would stop women who looked pregnant and talk to them. If I wasn't sure they were pregnant, I would just tell them I needed directions after stopping them and realizing, "Oh crap! I can't tell if you're really pregnant." Interviews were conducted face-to-face, online, over the phone, in airports, at malls, in coffee shops, and wherever else I saw a big belly or stroller headed my way.

- **I interviewed medical experts.** One of my favorite questions I'd ask the doctors when researching the book was, "What can't you say to a patient, but you've always wanted to say?" I felt it was important to talk to doctors so that the information in this book would be accurate and helpful.

- **I included letters, tips, and feedback from readers.** I love second editions because they are so much stronger than the first. For this edition, I used all the feedback, letters, tips, and stories from the people who have been there and done it. This book is more balanced, deeper, and better.

- **I reviewed relevant materials.** If you walked into my office, you would think that I'm either a little too excited about having another baby or writing a book. Anything I could get my hands on, I would read. One of the coolest things was getting daily Google Alerts. You can sign up for alerts at Google and then get stories from around the world that include relevant keywords you've submitted. Every morning I read about the news with the keywords "Expectant Father" and "Pregnant Woman."

ABOUT THE TIPS AND STORIES
As you flip through the pages, you'll read a tip and a story. The majority of the stories you'll read are verbatim, from the

mouths of the people sharing them. Some tips and stories were submitted via my website (www.HelpMeHarlan.com) and others were gathered via interviews. If I interviewed someone and didn't have a pad and paper, I would later write the stories down in the voice of the person relaying the story. When attributing stories, I used the name of the person sharing the story and the age and gender or genders of that person's child or children. A small percentage of the contributors asked me to change their first name to protect their identity. If a tip or story was submitted using an alias, I would assign a name to the story submitted. The goal was to create a free-flowing dialogue where people could share *whatever* was on their minds. I've found that this method of sharing is successful in allowing contributors to feel completely at ease.

ABOUT THE CONTENT AND WORD CHOICES

Pregnancy and birth are extremely personal topics. I get it. The choices you make are the best choices for you. To reflect the personal nature of this experience, I did my best to be objective. I included information about natural birth, home birth, hospital birth, doulas, midwives, doctors, epidural, no pain medication, nursing, formula feeding, and other issues about which people have very strong beliefs. I did my very best to offer a balanced view of the expectant father experience. This book isn't about me forcing one belief or practice on an individual, but reporting the experience in a manner that shows all differing points of view. I avoided using the words "husbands" and "wives" and instead used "partners." I often used the word "caregiver" instead of "doctor." I frequently used "birth location" instead of "hospital." If you have a particular point of view and would like me to consider it for future editions, please send it to me by emailing me at Harlan@helpmeharlan .com or via www.DadsExpectingToo.com. I know this is a sensitive area and want to make sure all sides and all voices are represented.

NOPE, THIS ISN'T A MEDICAL GUIDE

I'm not a doctor, but this book has been medically reviewed. It's also been read and recommended by caregivers over the years. While this book has medical information, it is not a medical guide. If you have questions, please consult your caregiver. This book may help you to come up with questions and be more comfortable asking questions, but any concerns you have should be addressed by a medical professional.

THE SECOND OF MORE EDITIONS

As you go through this experience, please share with me your thoughts and feelings. If you like something, let me know. If you don't like something, let me know. If there's something missing in here, please let me know. If you think I've gotten something wrong, let me know. You can swear at me and call me names, but please make sure there's a suggestion after you're done with your verbal beatdown. Please email me at Harlan@helpmeharlan.com or via Harlan @DadsExpectingToo.com or via www.DadsExpectingToo .com. Thank you so much for the support. I look forward to hearing from you.

WE ARE PIONEERS...

When my mom went into labor, my dad was given a chair in the expectant fathers' waiting room. My dad didn't hold her hand, comfort her through labor, encourage her to push, hold her leg, cut the cord, hear my first cry, or document the first moments of my life with multiple video devices. He wasn't allowed inside the room.

Fast-forward thirty-three years and I was front and center in the middle of the action. I saw it all, heard it all, and tried to capture it all on a camera and cell phone. Today, expectant fathers are no longer stuck in the waiting room—we are in the trenches watching it unfold in real time. From the moment the pee hits the stick, we are on call, engaged, immersed, and involved in childbirth like no generation of men that has come before us.

We are pregnancy pioneers.

Unlike the sisterhood of women who have been sharing pregnancy stories through the ages, there is no such brotherhood. But now, that's all about to change... .

1

THE FIRST FEW WEEKS...

Shock, Joy, Surprise, and Things You'll Want to Do When the Baby Is Born

Tip #1
THE MAGIC URINE: The Day We Officially Lose Control

THE TIP:
You can take a pregnancy test yourself, but only hers counts.

THE STORY:
The first four tests she took were all positive, but the indicator strips were extremely light. That's when I took a fifth test to act as a control test to make sure the results were accurate. She laughed at first but generally thought I was an idiot for doing so. She stood next to me as I took the test (she turned away when I peed). After dipping the stick,

my wife watched as the indicator light revealed the results. As predicted, the results were a bright negative. For some reason, I had to test it. I just couldn't believe it.

—*Scott, daughter, twenty-three months*

***

The lack of control begins with her pee.

My wife hoarded her urine—she insisted it was too early to take a pregnancy test and refused to pee on a stick for me. I insisted she share her pee. While I agreed it was too early to get accurate results, taking a pregnancy test is too much fun to pass up. How many times in our lives would we get to do this?

She explained that she didn't want to be disappointed if the test was negative like the previous month's round of testing. We agreed that a negative result was the most likely outcome and decided we wouldn't be disappointed because it was so early. She handed me some of her possibly pregnant urine to test—just for fun. She then quickly took it back and dipped the pregnancy test stick. We huddled around the urine-soaked magic wand, waiting.

Pregnancy tests detect the pregnancy hormone hCG. hCG begins to be produced when a fertilized egg implants in the uterus—about six days after conception—and then continues to increase during pregnancy. Most pregnancy tests give the most accurate results once hCG reaches high enough levels in the urine to be detected, about one week after a missed period. Early pregnancy tests can be used to tell if you're pregnant up to five days before a missed period.

Once we dipped the stick and waited two minutes, we saw what appeared to be the faintest blue line. The line was so faint it almost wasn't there. It definitely wasn't negative, but it was barely positive. We turned it, we put it under a bright light, dipped it one more time to see if it changed—still, the results were unclear.

Fast-forward fifteen minutes, and I returned home from the drugstore with three deluxe digital home pregnancy tests. She peed again, we huddled again, and then the word *pregnant* flashed on the screen. We took another test and it said *not pregnant*. She then took another digital test from a different manufacturer, and the results flashed *pregnant*. We figured two flashing pregnant sticks meant that she was really pregnant.

After more research, I learned that tests *rarely* ever give false positives. (hCG levels can vary from day to day, which can make someone have a positive test one day and then a negative test the next.) So a positive result normally means

PREGNANCY Q & A

QUESTION: Number of pregnancy tests she took?
ANSWER: Around three or four.

QUESTION: How long it took for her to get pregnant?
ANSWER: About two months.

QUESTION: Where it happened (location)?
ANSWER: We think conception happened at home on the middle landing of the (carpeted) stairs the night after we saw the movie *The Break-Up*.

that you can be pretty sure she is pregnant. My wife took another test with her morning pee, and we were 100 percent positive. Four cheap tests and three digital tests later (a total of $75 worth of sticks), we finally believed she was pregnant.

This was the moment I lost control. As a man, I didn't even have control over the test—that's how little control we have from day one. But as I would learn, the sooner I accepted the lack of control and yielded to the universe, the sooner I could get comfortable with the uncomfortable and enjoy this wild ride.

THE BOTTOM LINE:

Put your urine away and go with her flow. There's no controlling the future even if you pee on a control stick.

Tip #2
REACTING TO THE NEWS: It Doesn't Quite Seem Real Yet

THE TIP:

The first few days are surreal; then normal life returns.

THE STORY:

We had been trying to get pregnant for eight months. The lack of control we had over our ability to conceive was a source of discomfort. The longer we tried, the more impatient we started to feel. By month four of trying to conceive, we knew we were doing everything in our power to become pregnant and that some of this process was just out of our control, so we started to release ourselves to the universe. We also switched from the pregnancy test with the lines to the test that had a smiley face as the positive indicator (the marketing got us—what would you rather see, a line or a smile?). This particular morning, we were both standing around the bathroom sink waiting for the test to reveal the answer. When the smiley face began to emerge, we just stared at it in disbelief. We gave it a couple more minutes to turn negative, but it stayed positive. We couldn't believe it worked. Once the disbelief subsided, there was happiness, then a fear that it wouldn't stick (some of our friends had miscarried), then excitement that it happened, followed by relief that we could conceive. It's funny; the month we got pregnant was the month we relied on the least amount of science to get pregnant.

—*Mike, son, three months*

***

Congratulations! You are now an expectant father. You got someone pregnant. Feels good, right?

You might be shocked, happy, surprised, fearful, joyous, disappointed, relieved, panicked, regretful, ecstatic, numb, or full of pride. Or you might not know what to feel.

> He found out Christmas morning. I put the pregnancy test in his stocking. He kept looking at me, confused and surprised, saying, "Really?"
>
> —*Cathy, sons, four months and three and a half*

Once the initial shock passes and your emotions settle down, life might not seem all that different for you. You're not the one with morning sickness. As a man, you know something big is happening, but until you can see it, touch it, or hear it, you can have a hard time processing pregnancy and what's happening. A man needs to hear the heartbeat, see the ultrasound, and feel the baby kick to grab onto the fact that things are changing. It can take months for it to hit you. I'm convinced that pregnancy lasts forty weeks because it takes a guy a good five months to believe it and another four months to get the furniture delivered.

On the other side of the bed is your expectant partner. She is consumed with change. All her energy is channeled into the pregnancy from the moment the test turns positive. She is hyperfocused. Once the test turns positive, she'll go online and find a pregnancy group. She'll buy pregnancy books. She'll download apps. She'll subscribe to pregnancy magazines, order catalogs (for the baby's room), shop for maternity clothing, register for baby stuff, clean the house, and do anything else that can help her start preparing for the big event.

In the meantime, your life changes far less during the first few months. You'll do things to prepare for the baby, but it's not quite real yet. If you've been engaged, it's kind of like right after you propose to her. The moment the ring goes on her finger, she's off to the races planning the wedding. It's total immersion—books, magazines, planners, conversations with friends,

> We had just returned from a week's vacation and pretty much knew we were preggers, and it was *very* unplanned. I just came out of the bathroom that morning crying and holding a very positive test stick. After I crawled back into the bed next to him, he said, "I've never been so scared, excited, and proud all at the same time…My boys can swim!!!"
>
> —Misti, daughter, twenty-four months

and anything else she can consume to help her with what's next. Meanwhile, most men aren't in the same place at the same time. Once a guy sees his bride walking down the aisle, he starts to get excited because he knows that it's real. It's not that we don't care. We're just programmed differently.

The challenge here is that a woman might misinterpret your actions (or lack thereof) as uncaring. She might think that you are not as happy if you're not doing as much as she is to get ready for the baby. So the best way to connect is to take an active role. She won't force you—you have to be willing and proactive.

One of the easiest ways to feel connected and involved is to read the week-by-week pregnancy updates with your partner. (You can find them in this book and on the Dad's Expecting Too Tracker at www.DadsExpectingToo.com.) The first twelve weeks of pregnancy are some of the most remarkable and dramatic weeks of development. If you keep up with what's happening, you will be involved, engaged, and more connected. You'll get excited when you read about each week's changes. And when you're excited and connected, you won't have to work so hard to convince her that you're part of this process.

THE BOTTOM LINE:

Once you meet your new baby, you'll know this is real. For now, check out pages 75–94 for a week-by-week guide to what's happening inside her belly and pretend it's real (because it's real).

Tip #3
SHARING THE NEWS: Who, When, and How to Tell

THE TIP:
When you're not yet telling people and someone asks, it's really hard to lie about it.

THE STORY:
Our agreement was that if somebody asked, then we would tell. When somebody asks if you are pregnant, and you are, you can't help but hesitate, and they know if you say no that you're lying. So we had planned to tell our family first at Thanksgiving. My wife has a close group of grade school friends, and one of them had a baby shower. The whole time, she dodged the topic. She even snuck in a glass of orange juice while everybody else was drinking mimosas. Finally as it was time to leave, some random coworker of the hostess approaches my wife and blurts out, "I noticed you weren't drinking. Are you pregnant?" The secret was out. My parents flew in for Thanksgiving, and we had everybody over for dinner. Before we ate, I gave a toast to thank God for all his blessings over the past year. I closed the prayer by asking God to watch over us as we welcome the newest member of our family next July. After a couple of seconds, everybody understood what I was trying to say, and lots of noise and congrats followed. My usually non-emotional father even started to tear up.

—*Kevin, three months pregnant*

***

You might want to shout to the world "I am going to be a father!" You might be tempted to post it on Facebook, tweet it, or blog about it. You might want to tell your coworkers, friends, and neighbors. However you do it, you might want to wait until week eleven or twelve. Yes, proclaiming you're expecting makes it real, but it also makes it public. Why is that a problem? For some couples, it's not. For others, it's better to wait.

WHY WAIT?

The first couple of months are the most unpredictable. It's the riskiest time during the pregnancy. That's why people will wait until twelve weeks into the pregnancy to share the news with the world. After the twelve-week checkup, the chances of miscarriage go dramatically down. Telling before twelve weeks means that if the pregnancy should end unexpectedly, you'll have to explain to all the people who received your Facebook update that you are no longer expecting. And this personal process isn't something everyone wants to share publicly. Waiting to tell protects you and your partner from having to explain yourself should something not go as planned.

> There are so many celebratory events that occur in your life that you tell everyone. This one was so uniquely special because it was a secret between us.
>
> —Don, sons, twenty-two months and four months

If your pregnant partner wants to tell more people than you originally agreed to tell (sharing the news with one friend can turn into five friends), try not to make her feel bad for sharing. She might need more support than she originally thought she would need. Just make sure she tells you who she tells. This way, if she tells a friend and that friend tells your friend, you will know that your friend knows, and you won't have to lie if he asks you about it. Assume that if she tells her friend, that friend will tell her significant other, even if she forbids her from telling (no one can keep it a secret).

WHY WAIT?

You may not want your employer to know. Not all employers react favorably to an employee having a baby. Once you share the news, word will travel fast. The reality is that having a baby can be disruptive to work (especially for women). There's something to be said about waiting and telling employers until you have to let them know. Having your significant other tell them early doesn't do anything other than cause her boss to start wondering right away what is going to happen to her desire to work after she gives birth.

If she's the boss, then she can do whatever the hell she wants (perks of being a boss).

WHY WAIT?

You are superstitious. You think that telling will affect the pregnancy. I don't believe that superstition will change the outcome, although I'm not going to commit to this (call me superstitious). What's so interesting about superstition is that these rules we

> With one of our pregnancies, we told too soon, and it unfortunately ended in a miscarriage. Waiting until after the first trimester is always recommended—now we know why. It saves a whole lot of heartache that can happen if people still think you're pregnant and you aren't anymore.
>
> —Patrick, father of five, expecting number six

live by have no rational foundation. But when dealing with the unknown and having so little control over the process, we tend to make rules. Superstitions are just about control. That's one reason you'll find so many people are so superstitious when it comes to having a baby.

HOW TO SHARE

Facebook, Twitter, Pinterest, Tumblr, and other social networks make it easy to share intimate details about your life with family, friends, and that kid you sat next to in eighth grade. It also makes it easy to hurt people's feelings or share too much with too many people. Your aunt in California might not be on Facebook. So when her granddaughter tells her that you're having a baby and her granddaughter heard about it first on Facebook, your aunt might feel left out. Make sure that the people you want to know the news hear it straight from you, instead of via a retweet or through someone who has no business sharing this news. Also, if something unexpected should happen, you might not want to share that news with *everyone* who has access to your social networks.

THE ODD RESPONSE

When you share the news, people will say stupid things. Expect it. For example, childhood friends, single and unattached friends, jealous siblings, parents, and unstable relatives often say inappropriate and dumb things. For example, when you say, "I've got some exciting news. WE'RE EXPECTING A BABY!!!" They may respond with:

- "Is it yours?"
- "Why, why, why? (shaking head)"

- "Ever hear of condoms?"
- "They'll let anyone be a dad!"
- "You are so screwed!"
- "Have you heard of the pull-out method?"
- "You keeping it?"
- "What the hell are you thinking?"
- "Does she know?"
- "Aren't you a virgin?"
- "Why'd you do that, dumbass!"

As a first-time expectant father, any feedback other than what you expect can put you on the defensive or on the attack (you might get pissed). Recognize that the reactions are more about the people offering them than you. For example, the news might make a childhood friend who is single feel threatened, a parent feel old (mom or dad is going to be a grandma or grandpa), a sibling feel jealous, or a boss feel concerned. Their reactions are rarely about you or your parenting skills. These stupid comments are a reflection of other people's insecurities. If something bothers you, tell them their response makes you uncomfortable ("uncomfortable" is a nonconfrontational word that says it all). At least this way they can have a chance to explain their poor choice of words.

THE BOTTOM LINE:

Some people, whether intentional or not, will make stupid comments.

THE TIP:

We used a midwife for both pregnancies. If I hadn't had a vasectomy, we'd use one again.

THE STORY:

The midwife was already part of my wife's gynecologist's office, so it just worked out. I didn't know what a midwife did, but my wife filled me in. Some appointments were with the doctor and some were with the midwife. Both of them were good about asking us how we were doing. There were only two professionals in the practice, so I got to know everyone, even the secretary. (I went to all the appointments.) It was a small and friendly place. The midwife was kind of a mentor during the pregnancy and delivery. She would ask me what I wanted to do and then offer me instructions. When my wife, who wanted to have a natural delivery (no medication), had to get an epidural and Pitocin because her labor was not moving along, the midwife was there to reassure us. We used the same doctor and midwife for our second baby.

—*Jim, daughter, two months, son, three*

Some doctors can have a more clinical and "just the facts" style. Our midwife answered all the questions and took time with us at each appointment.

—*Mike, son, twelve months*

✳✳✳

A midwife is not a woman who fills in for your wife when she's pregnant—that would be called a mistress and that's just plain wrong. Just wanted to clear that up. As for delivering this kid, you and your partner have options. You can have an ob-gyn, a family doctor, or a midwife deliver the baby. You can have it at home, in a hospital, in a bathtub, on the floor, or hanging upside down (not sure how that works). So what are your options?

THE DOCTOR

Most women use an ob-gyn as their primary caregiver. If you're thinking about a natural delivery or birth outside of the hospital, a family physician might be the right fit. Sometimes, the ob-gyn who has treated your partner in the past might not be the best person to handle the pregnancy. Some doctors might do everything but deliveries (not all doctors in ob-gyn practices deliver).

If your partner experiences a high-risk pregnancy, her regular ob-gyn might not be the best fit—you may need a specialist. A doctor who prefers medically assisted births might not be a good fit for someone who wants a non-medicated, natural birth. Likewise, a woman who wants a medically assisted birth might not want a doctor who encourages a more holistic approach. There are also issues like the size of the practice, location of the practice, where she wants to deliver (hospital, birthing center, home), and if insurance offers you the freedom to pick and choose your doctor. (Some doctors might be out-of-network and therefore much more expensive.)

Your caregiver's personality is an important factor to consider. You and your partner need to feel comfortable and confident with her care. If the doctor is impatient and dismissive, find someone else. Also, get to know the other doctors in the practice. There is no guarantee that who she sees before the birth will be present during the delivery. This might freak her out (and you). It's not uncommon for someone else to do the delivery. Make sure to meet the other doctors (just in case). My wife's primary doctor didn't deliver either of our kids. The other doctors who did the delivery were awesome. We thought that knowing in advance who would deliver the baby was a big deal, but turned out not to matter—shocking, I know. We literally met the delivering doctor an hour before our daughter was born and loved our experience. When it came time for my son's delivery, my wife's doctor was at his daughter's birthday party. So the doctor on call delivered my son. This doctor was amazing too. Good practices don't keep bad doctors.

When it comes to the number of doctors in the practice, size can matter. Some women find large practices less personal and are uncomfortable with not knowing who will show up on the day she goes into labor. Some may find a smaller practice lacking in resources and support services. There are pros and cons associated with both.

Note: You should be able to ask your partner's caregiver questions without feeling like you're being annoying (and to speak up if you feel uncomfortable). When choosing the doctor, she should be completely comfortable and make sure that you're comfortable. Discuss your birth plan (see Tip #73) and make sure the doctor's style and bedside manner are a good match.

THE MIDWIFE

A midwife isn't a doctor or a wife (although she can be married). There are two kinds of midwives in the United

States: certified nurse-midwives and direct-entry midwives. According to the American College of Nurse-Midwives (ACNM), "Certified nurse-midwives are registered nurses who have graduated from a nurse-midwifery education program accredited by the ACNM Division of Accreditation (DOA) and have passed a national certification examination to receive the professional designation of certified nurse-midwife." A direct-entry midwife does not have the nursing training and cannot prescribe medication. A direct-entry midwife can also be called a certified professional midwife (if certified with the North American Registry of Midwives [NARM]).

A midwife approaches pregnancy differently than many doctors. The midwife's approach is one of mind and body. A midwife will speak to the needs of the expectant mother (and father) on a personal, spiritual, and medical level. She wants you and your partner to be completely at ease and connected with the care and process.

Some doctors work with midwives. If you're worried about a midwife taking over your role as a labor partner, don't be. Most midwives will encourage you to be as large a part of the process as you want to be. A midwife is definitely an option worth exploring. When my son was born, the hospital had a midwife on-site. This was my first interaction with a midwife, and she was amazing. She asked us what we wanted to happen before, during, and after delivery. She offered suggestions. She had suggestions on how to make my wife more comfortable. She had ideas of what should happen after the baby was delivered. Our midwife was a comfort. While you might be an expert getting her pregnant, it's helpful to have another set of eyes and easier to get the baby out of her.

If working with an ob-gyn, have your partner ask the doctor how he or she feels about having a doula or midwife participating in labor and delivery. Some doctors may have strong reactions (pro or con). It helps to know how the ob-gyn feels about having someone else involved in the procedure before delivery so there won't be any surprises. Ask if the hospital or birthing facility has a midwife on staff.

THE DOULA

A doula is a birth coach, advocate, partner, teammate, and a trusted ally throughout the pregnancy. She may work with your partner extensively prior to delivery or just meet with her briefly and show up when your partner goes into labor. A doula typically focuses on the comfort of the mother by doing things like offering an explanation of what's going on during labor and delivery, offering words of encouragement, rubbing her back during labor, or even holding the mother's hand. Like a midwife, the doula wants partners to be part of the experience.

While a doula doesn't deliver the baby, the doula is there for the delivery with the doctor or midwife. The doula knows the playbook and can offer tips, strategies, and insights that will help execute the birth plan. There is research that points to a reduced rate of C-sections, episiotomies, and complications with doula-assisted births. The doula is focused on creating the most comfortable, healthy, and empowering experience for the mother *and* father. When investigating a doula, visit DONA International at www.dona.org. A doula can cost between $300 to $1,200, depending on her level of involvement.

THE BOTTOM LINE:

You can't control labor and delivery, but you can control who is in the room with you. Put together the best team to help you and your partner have the most comfortable delivery.

Tip #5
WHERE TO HAVE IT: Birthing Centers, Hospitals, Homes, Cars, Cabs, Sidewalks…

THE TIP:

Having the birth in a hospital setting is just one option.

THE STORY:

After having two children in a hospital setting, we weighed the risks and we decided to have our third one at home—it was a dramatic difference. As a chiropractor, I've held a very naturalistic philosophy around health and wellness. It is beyond me that we treat the birth process as a medical condition. When I looked at the history of women giving birth, most births did not happen in a hospital. I've always thought of the hospital as a place for someone who is sick. It didn't make sense from my point of view to have another hospital birth. At home, it was far more relaxed, no rushing, and it all happened at a natural time. If a problem came up during the delivery, the doctor would have seen it coming. There was a medical van waiting in the driveway just in case. The birth went off without a hitch.

—*Stuart, daughters, nine, six, and two*

***

She can give birth in your bathtub or your bed at home. You can also do it in a hospital, at a birthing center, or some place in between (airplanes, buses, and cabs).

After going through labor and delivery two times, I'm still a hospital birth kind of guy. The idea of unexpected complications makes a hospital setting comfortable for my wife and me. That said, a hospital is a medical center—no question about it. It's not home. It's sterile. It's medical. There are nurses poking in and out, staff running around, and doctors coming and going. Then there may be visiting hours, a checkout time, and other rules and regulations. There are lots of people and different personalities to manage. As helpful as we found the attention and constant care, other people I spoke with found it intrusive.

Considering that a hospital birth is the most common place to deliver, the idea of *not* giving birth at a hospital might freak you out (or your family). If your pregnant partner wants to explore other options, don't freak out. (Your family physician may also be qualified to perform deliveries. Home births will often be facilitated by a family physician.) Do some research and get a better handle on it.

Whatever you decide, talk to people who have done it before and ask about their birth plan. The birth plan includes things like whether she wants medication, who you want to deliver the baby (ob-gyn, midwife, family doctor), and postpartum care (what happens after the baby is born). Once you know what you want, find the right venue to have the baby (see Tip #73 for information on birth plans).

BIRTHING CENTERS

A birthing center is the closest thing to home without being

COMFORT IS SUBJECTIVE

If your partner wants a medical team down the hall "just in case," a hospital birth is the place for you (and me).

at home. Birthing centers can be attached to a hospital, next to a hospital, or freestanding. They are typically for women interested in having natural births who have a low risk of complications. Care is most frequently provided by a certified nurse-midwife, a direct-entry midwife, or a nurse. Birth centers do not perform any "routine" medical procedures. A fetal monitor and IV are not necessarily part of a birthing center birth, but they can be available. By doing away with most high-tech equipment and routine procedures, labor and birth remain a natural and personal process. If you are interested in delivering at a birthing center, make sure it is accredited by the Commission for the Accreditation of Birth Centers. Accredited birthing centers must have affiliated doctors at a nearby hospital in case problems arise with the mom or baby. For information about birthing centers, you can check out www.birthcenters.org.

QUESTIONS YOU SHOULD ASK WHEN DECIDING WHERE TO HAVE THE KID:

- How close is the facility?
- Does the hospital offer birthing classes? How many? Cost?
- What kind of paperwork needs to be completed?

- Will my medical information be here? Do we need to bring a copy?
- Are there birth balls, music players, or other amenities?
- What types of medication are available?
- What is the procedure for administering anesthesia? Are epidurals available?
- Is anesthesia available twenty-four hours?
- Is there a neonatal intensive care unit on-site?
- Does the hospital encourage natural labor or induced labor (using Pitocin)?
- How is labor monitored (type of fetal monitoring devices)?
- Is this a teaching hospital with residents?
- What are the rates of induction, episiotomy, epidurals, C-sections, and forceps-assisted and vacuum-assisted births?
- Are doulas available?
- Are midwives available?
- What is the philosophy of the birthing center or hospital?
- Who ensures the birth plan is followed? Procedures?
- Can we take photos and/or videos during the birth?
- What are the visiting hours and rules regarding number of visitors at one time?
- What are the C-section procedures? Can Dad be there? Doula? Is baby given to Mom immediately?
- Following labor, is the room private?
- Can people stay overnight? Average length of stay (usually longer after C-section)?
- Is a lactation consultant available?
- Does baby stay in Mom's room or in the nursery?

THE BOTTOM LINE:
The best place to give birth is where you and your partner can be comfortable, calm, and get the best care—covered by insurance is a nice bonus too.

Tip #6
HOW TO PAY FOR IT: Now Is a Good Time to Check Your Insurance

THE TIP:
Discuss coverage for the baby with a health insurance agent. Saving a few hundred dollars today could cost you tomorrow.

THE STORY:
My wife was working full-time before she got pregnant. She had much better health benefits than I did. She was planning on quitting once she had the baby. We were all set to put the baby on her policy because it was hundreds of dollars cheaper and a better all-around policy. Our insurance agent advised us not to be so quick to put the baby under her coverage. If he was on my wife's policy and she quit her job, then both she and the baby would need insurance. If the baby had some sort of birth defect, getting insurance could be more difficult. Putting him under my policy meant that no matter what, he would be covered.

—Danny, son, twenty-one months

✳✳✳

Did you know maternity coverage isn't always part of insurance? (I think I just heard someone scream.)

If you find out that your partner is pregnant and not covered by insurance, there's some good news. A lot of hospitals, labs, and healthcare providers will offer substantial discounts to individuals paying out-of-pocket. Even if you have insurance, always ask about discounts for out-of-pocket bills. Assistance might also be available through the state or federal government (depending on your level of income). Should you ever get a bill, ask the provider for a discount. When we were charged a lot for genetic testing (see Tip #12), the lab took off 30 percent just because I asked. All you have to do is ask, and they'll typically give you a break on most medical bills (not just genetic testing).

Assuming you have coverage, get familiar with your policy's rules and regulations. If you have a health insurance agent, give him or her a call. If you want to call the insurance provider directly, that works too. You're going to want to find out what your coverage includes so you can make the right moves. Some insurance companies require that you notify them immediately after finding out that you're expecting. Others want to know when you check into the

WARNING

If changing coverage, inquire about waiting periods. Some health insurance providers have waiting periods before maternity coverage kicks in. You might have to wait twelve months until maternity coverage takes effect, which means you're effectively on your own if birth control fails.

GREAT INSURANCE INFORMATION

With the recent passage and implementation of the Affordable Care Act, health insurance is changing faster than books can be printed and downloaded. For the latest info visit: www.healthcare.gov/.

hospital for delivery. There may be rules that must be followed to ensure coverage (or you could end up with penalties and bills).

When it comes to method of delivery, type of care, and location of care provided, make sure you know your options. It's a bad idea to begin investigating these questions after the baby is born or while passing time during labor because…well, because that's just not responsible (although never investigating would be even less responsible). Find out things like the number of ultrasounds covered by your plan, whether your hospital is in-network, and what kind of prenatal care is provided as soon as possible. Contact your healthcare provider or health insurance agent and go over the questions listed below. When dealing with insurance providers, always get information in writing (email works). In addition, make sure you get the name of the person you speak with and their identification number. Keep a notebook and title it "Pregnancy Insurance Archives" or "PIA." Should you end up in a disagreement with your insurance provider, having names and ID numbers will prove invaluable.

QUESTIONS YOU SHOULD ASK:

- What does your health care coverage include?

LOST YOUR COVERAGE?

If you lose your job, change jobs, or lose coverage during pregnancy, investigate COBRA (Consolidated Omnibus Budget Reconciliation Act) insurance. COBRA gives workers and their families who lose their health benefits the right to choose to continue group health benefits provided by their group health plan for limited periods of time under certain circumstances such as voluntary or involuntary job loss, reduction in the number of hours worked, transition between jobs, death, divorce, and other life events. Qualified individuals may be required to pay the entire premium for coverage, up to 102 percent of the cost of the plan. COBRA generally requires that group health plans sponsored by employers with twenty or more employees in the prior year offer employees and their families the opportunity for a temporary extension of health coverage (called continuation coverage) in certain instances where coverage under the plan would otherwise end. It could cost a little more, but it's a short-term solution that can save you in the long run.

(Source: www.dol.gov/dol/topic/health-plans/cobra.htm)

- What kind of prenatal tests are covered (and how many ultrasounds)?

- Is preauthorization required for any prenatal or maternal care?
- What is your deductible (the amount you will be responsible for paying before the insurance company begins to pay the bills)?
- What percentage of the bill will you have to pay? (You might have to pay a percentage of the cost based on the type of plan you have. Twenty percent can be a lot to budget for.)
- Is the doctor or midwife part of the plan? (Not all doctors are in-network.)
- Do they cover midwives, doulas, or other services?
- Does coverage include birthing centers and home births?
- Do you need to contact your health insurance provider when admitted into the hospital?
- If you need a longer stay due to medical issues, what is the procedure?
- Does your coverage include a private room or semi-private room? Cost to upgrade?
- What hospitals are in-network and out-of-network? (In-network hospitals have agreements with the insurance provider; out-of-network hospitals are not always covered as thoroughly and can be more complicated.)
- Do they cover cord blood storage or offer a discount?
- IMPORTANT: What is the procedure to add coverage for the newborn? (Generally this has to be done within thirty days of the birth.)
- What does the coverage include once the baby is born?
- What are the rules regarding a pediatrician who is either in- or out-of-network?
- Is lactation counseling covered?

- Does coverage include circumcision? What about care once the baby leaves the hospital?

QUESTIONS TO DISCUSS WITH YOUR PARTNER:

- Will the baby be on your policy or her policy? (If she's going to stop working and you're on her policy, make sure you have coverage and that the baby has coverage. Set it up *now*.)
- Do you have a pediatrician in mind? Is he or she in your network?
- What vaccines do you want the baby to receive?
- Do you want to do cord blood storage? (See Tip #77.)

PREGNANCY Q & A
QUESTION: Any medical surprises?
ANSWER: The doctor mentioned my uterus was a little big and I could be having twins. We don't know yet. We are waiting for the first ultrasound, and since our insurance only covers one, we want to have it later so that we can find out the sex at the same time. My husband is very excited and hopes for twins. I hope he won't be disappointed.
—Tiffany, seven weeks pregnant

KEY INSURANCE TERMS

HMO: Health Maintenance Organization. An HMO consists of an organization of healthcare providers (doctors and hospitals) that offer their services at a fixed price and are contracted with an insurance company. The rules and restrictions of HMO plans can be limiting. Your primary care physician will manage your health care and must be a member of the HMO. This means you might need a new doctor in the network (if your current doctor isn't in-network). In order to see a specialist, your primary care physician must be the one to refer you, but you can always go out-of-network and pay additional fees.

PPO: Preferred Provider Organization. A PPO consists of a more loosely organized group of doctors and hospitals that have a contractual relationship with an insurance company. A PPO gives you the flexibility to see whichever doctor you choose. You have the option to select an out-of-network physician, but you will have to pay more out-of-pocket. You also don't need a referral to see a specialist. PPOs cost more than HMOs, but many people choose them because they are far less restrictive.

IN-NETWORK PROVIDER: a care provider who has an agreement with the insurance provider.

OUT-OF-NETWORK PROVIDER: a care provider who doesn't have an agreement with the insurance provider.

PREMIUM: the amount you pay for coverage.

DEDUCTIBLE: the amount you have to pay before the insurance company picks up the bill.

MEDICAID: government-subsidized coverage for low-income families.

LIFE OR DISABILITY INSURANCE

Chances are you will live a full life. But there's always the most remote chance that you might get hit by a bus (while checking your email on your phone to see if she's in labor yet). If you do meet a bus or some unpredictable and highly unlikely demise, it's comforting to think that you will still be able to provide for your family. Life insurance and disability insurance are *not* about you. They're about the people who rely on you financially and emotionally. The last thing anyone needs during a stressful emotional time is financial distress. And that's what insurance is for. Some people don't want to get life or disability insurance because it implies death or tragedy, and some people hate the idea of death or tragedy, but it's about enabling those you love to maintain their lifestyle.

The general rule is that you want enough insurance to enable your family to maintain their lifestyle and take care of financial obligations in the future (mortgage, child care, loans, car payments). How much insurance you'll need to get varies, but get it. Talk to a qualified agent or financial planner to discuss your individual needs. You might be thinking that the last thing you can afford is life insurance, but once you check it out, you'll be surprised at how inexpensive it can be. Assuming you're in relatively good health, we're talking less than a monthly telephone bill. And while you're talking about life insurance, look into disability insurance. Disability insurance replaces your income if you become disabled and can't work (talk to your agent for details). Here's one way to think about it— how long do you go on vacation when you take one? Not more than a couple weeks—because you need to work. You can't afford to take more time. Imagine being disabled and not being able to work for months or years. Scary? That's the value of disability insurance. While you never want to use insurance, it's comforting to know that if something should happen to you, your family will be taken care of.

THE BOTTOM LINE:
If your doctor requires cash, check to see if there's an ATM in the delivery room. If you find an ATM in the delivery room, you're probably in an ATM lobby and should get to the nearest hospital.

Tip #7
FEEDING YOUR PREGNANT PARTNER: Keep Your Fingers Far Away from Her Mouth...

THE TIP:
Don't question cravings—just get her what she wants.

THE STORY:
I got constant food cravings. The cravings can be weird. With my first, I couldn't get enough orange juice. With the second, it's been chocolate. There's no rational reason—it just happens. Not only did I get cravings, but food aversions. During the first trimester, I was sick or nauseous and I couldn't stomach eating meat. I couldn't prepare it. I couldn't be around it. I couldn't look at it. Chicken was the worst. The sight of all meat absolutely repulsed me. I'm telling you, raw meat was disgusting, gross, nasty, and horrible. I ate peanut butter and jelly and grilled cheese

sandwiches for weeks. My husband didn't ask me to explain, and that's a good thing, because I couldn't explain it. He just went with the flow. Once I hit twenty-five weeks, it all started to go away. A few weeks later, I was in full force eating steak, chicken, and all those things I loved. It's not logical or rational—gosh no, but it's just how it was.

SEVEN FOODS TO FEED HER

1. Whole grains
2. Beans
3. Salmon
4. Eggs
5. Colorful fruit
6. Leafy greens
7. Greek yogurt

—Denise, daughter, twenty-one months, thirty-two weeks pregnant

BONUS TIP:
Get her EXACTLY what she wants. Do not deviate!

Don't try to understand—just go with it. Last pregnancy, she wanted orange soda and gyros every day for a month, and she *hates* gyros. Won't even look at them now. This time it's orange sherbet and grilled cheese sandwiches with sweet pickles. Gotta be gherkins.

—Patrick, expecting baby number six

THE STORY:
During my first pregnancy, I was craving green Hi-C (ecto cooler if you were a kid in the 80s). He was gone for over an hour, and when he came home he had a packet of lime Kool-Aid. I looked at it, then at him, and asked, "What is that?" He said, "Green Hi-C?" I said, "It's not! It's Kool-Aid!" I then proceeded to

WANT A HAPPY PREGNANT PARTNER?

Never, never, never tell her, "You are eating for two, not four."
—Moss, daughters, three and five

throw myself on my mattress and cry…
—*Jamie, sons, six and four, daughter, two*

***

If you are feeding your pregnant partner a chunk of blue cheese, raw sushi, undercooked bacon, cookie batter (with raw egg), and a glass of warm cow's milk direct from the udder (unpasteurized) moments after picking up the kitty litter box with your bare hands (the hands you're now feeding your partner with), throw down this book and scream, "STOP EATING!"

Now, wash your hands with soap and warm water immediately (scrub for at least thirty seconds) and continue reading.

Welcome back.

Your pregnant partner may get ravenously hungry. When the hunger hits, she must be fed. It's your job to satisfy her cravings. Be prepared to drive near or far. Get ready to heat, defrost, and prepare at all times. You are the 24/7 delivery man. It's your job to know what you can and can't feed her when the craving hits. Problem foods include: undercooked meats, deli meats (unless heated to the point where they're steaming), unpasteurized cheese (never blue cheese), and

If you want to have a happy relationship, NEVER eat the last bratwurst—NEVER.
—*Doug, daughter, three, son, three*

certain seafood (unless it's been cooked, *not* cured). When preparing fruits and vegetables, make sure they're washed extremely well. Also, keep cutlery, cutting boards, spatulas, plates, and dishes used to prepare raw foods far away from cooked foods (to prevent cross-contamination). If you're unsure how long a food has been in the fridge or if it's been sitting out too long, apply the "when in doubt, throw it out" rule.

When satisfying late-night cravings, keep food next to the bed (or in the

PREGNANCY TRIVIA
CATEGORY: Extra Calories Pregnant Women Need
QUESTION: How many additional calories does a pregnant woman need to consume on a daily basis?

    (a) 300 calories
    (b) 600 calories
    (c) 1,800 calories
    (d) 3,600 calories

(For the answer, see The Bottom Line.)

bed if it's a big enough bed). Sometimes your pregnant partner will be too uncomfortable to cook or prepare food for herself. If she does the cooking, this could be a tough situation for you. If you aren't used to the grocery store, get started or get groceries delivered.

A pregnant woman's palate changes minute by minute. So if you want to cook or prepare food for her, ask her what she wants and search for a recipe online. You'll find easy recipes that need very few ingredients. If she doesn't eat your cooking, don't be offended. She might see it or smell it and realize she can't bear to eat it. Don't take it personally if she vomits. If she vomits every single time,

CAFFEINE

When surprising her with a latte, make sure it's a decaf. Some studies show that drinking caffeine during pregnancy can harm the fetus. Other research suggests that small amounts of caffeine are safe. Talk to your doctor before encouraging her to drink caffeinated beverages during pregnancy. Caffeine can be found in many over-the-counter and prescription drugs.

your cooking might be the problem.

The easiest way to cook is to not cook—order in. If you do carry out, make sure you know what she should and shouldn't eat. This might mean asking the people on the phone lots of questions. (If you don't like being annoying, do your own cooking, because asking for special orders on the phone is annoying.) When ordering, tell them she's pregnant. You're not the first guy calling in a pregnant order. Make sure the cheese is pasteurized, ask if raw eggs are used in the Caesar salad dressing, and if ordering sushi, make sure the chef prepares your partner's cooked sushi far away from the raw fish (on a separate board with separate cutlery to avoid cross-contamination).

As for her cravings, they might not be so irrational. Pregnant women require more folic acid, iron, calcium, and water. While a prenatal vitamin should take care of the essentials (make sure she's taking prenatal vitamins), certain foods might be calling her name because the baby is craving essential nutrients. Orange juice, leafy greens, and dried beans are all rich in folic acid. A hunk of steak is rich in iron (make sure it's not pink). Ice cream is rich in calcium.

PREGNANT WOMEN'S GUIDE TO EATING MEAT

For a list of questionable foods, visit www.fda.gov/food/resourcesforyou/healtheducators/ucm081785.htm and check out www.mayoclinic.com/health/pregnancy-nutrition/PR00109. When it comes to food-borne illness, the big three concerns are *Listeria*, methylmercury, and *Toxoplasma gondii* (see the FDA website for full definitions). According to the CDC, pregnant women are about thirteen times more likely to get listeriosis than other healthy adults. Pregnant women are also at higher risk of being infected with toxoplasmosis (do not let her handle that cat litter and no rare meats).

- For whole cuts of meat (excluding poultry)
  - Cook to at least 145°F (63°C) as measured with a food thermometer placed in the thickest part of the meat, then allow the meat to rest for three minutes before carving or consuming.
- For ground meat (excluding poultry)
  - Cook to at least 160°F (71°C); ground meats do not require a rest time.
- For all poultry (whole cuts and ground)
  - Cook to at least 165°F (74°C), and for whole poultry, allow the meat to rest for three minutes before carving or consuming.
- For deli meat
  - Heat all meat until it is steaming.

(Source: www.cdc.gov/parasites/toxoplasmosis/gen_info/pregnant.html)

MEDICATIONS

If she gets sick during the pregnancy and she wants you to give her medication, check with your caregiver first. Some medications can pose a potential health risk. For example, nonsteroidal anti-inflammatory drugs (NSAIDs) like ibuprofen (Advil, Motrin), naproxen (Aleve), and aspirin (acetylsalicylate) can cause serious blood flow problems in the baby if used during the last three months of pregnancy (after twenty-eight weeks). Also, aspirin may increase the chance for bleeding problems in the mother and the baby during pregnancy or at delivery. Herbal tea seems harmless, but some teas are better than others. She must talk with her caregiver before taking any drugs or medicines while pregnant. If you look online for help, make sure it's a trusted source, but still talk to your doctor. Check out www .womenshealth.gov/publications/our-publications /fact-sheet/pregnancy-medicines.html.

THE BOTTOM LINE:

If she craves it, and it's not dangerous for her to eat it, then find it, cook it, or order it. Don't ask her questions about it. Especially not a trivia question about the number of additional calories she should be consuming—and the answer to the trivia question is: a) She needs three hundred additional calories a day.

(**Note:** This tip is meant to be read as a couple.)

THE TIP:
Being pregnant isn't a ticket to do whatever you want for nine months.

THE STORY:
I've witnessed it personally. It happens—usually with a woman who is high-maintenance to begin with. I have friends who joke about using their pregnancy to get their husbands to do things because they can. They'll talk about not wanting to do something and having their husbands clean, or cook, or do something because they just don't feel like doing it. I remember receiving a card when I got pregnant that said, "Congratulations, now you have an excuse to never lift a finger for nine months." Personally, I never flashed my Pregnancy Card—at least I don't think I have. I asked my husband to do things out of need, not because I was taking advantage of being pregnant. There were plenty of times I needed help. Eventually, a guy will just say forget it. It's a balancing act—I'm not one to abuse it.

—*Anne, daughter, one, son, three and a half*

***

Let me introduce you to the Pregnancy Card. It's magical, powerful, and something all pregnant women carry. The Pregnancy Card is her free pass. It's the excuse a pregnant woman can pull anytime, anywhere, and for whatever reason she sees fit. How it works: the other night, as she was getting ready to go to sleep, my wife asked me to get her cell phone charger from the kitchen. I was in bed, cozy, on the edge of sleep. She asked me again…only this time she pulled out the Pregnancy Card. She said, "Can you get my charger? I'm really tired and *pregnant*." And that's the Pregnancy Card. When it's pulled, a man must move and not ask questions.

As the author of a book about being an expectant father, I jumped out of bed, but paused to ask her a question. "Are you too tired to go downstairs or are you just pulling the Pregnancy Card?" Surprisingly, she admitted she was both. At seven weeks, she knew she shouldn't have used the Pregnancy Card for something I would have done without her whipping it out. She could have gotten what she wanted simply by flashing the Tired Wife Card.

And that brings me to the main reason why I suggested reading this tip with your partner—some pregnant women have been known to abuse the Pregnancy Card. Abuse is when a pregnant woman can do something for herself, but chooses to use her pregnancy to force her partner to take action. Asking you to do something isn't the problem. It's reminding you that she's pregnant when asking you to do something she can handle. The problem with abusing the Pregnancy Card is that when she really does need something, the card may become ineffective over time.

It's natural for women to test the power of the card early on, but absolute power can absolutely go to some pregnant women's heads. I know some pregnant women might think a man should do whatever she demands, but there is such a thing as abuse. It's the same as abusing food—a woman who uses her pregnancy as a license to eat everything and anything on the planet is a pregnant woman who will end up gaining a crazy amount of weight. A pregnant woman who uses her Pregnancy Card to boss and control her partner is a pregnant woman who might wear her man down and have him build up resentment. Once that baby is born, she will need you more than ever—encourage her to pace herself.

Sure, there are going to be times when basic functions will be harder for her than others, and we're always here to help. That's why it's so important to never abuse the Pregnancy Card.

THE BOTTOM LINE:

She can use but not abuse her Pregnancy Card. There is a credibility limit.

Looking for more great features to help you prep for your new arrival? Get the *Dad's Expecting Too* week-by-week pregnancy tracker, designed for dads and their partners, along with weekly updates about baby, your partner, and you at DadsExpectingToo.com.

***

To get the latest news, info, facts, and stats for new and expecting parents, follow @DadsExpecting on Twitter and check out the Dad's Expecting Facebook Page at www.Facebook.com /DadsExpecting.

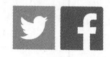

2

THE DOCTOR WILL SEE YOU NOW

Or Whoever Delivers Your Baby Will See You Now

Tip #9
YOUR FIRST GUYNE EXAM: Shake Hands with the Doctor (Then Wash)

THE TIP:
Shock and awe are the best words to describe the first doctor's visit.

THE STORY:
Going to the first visit with my wife wasn't optional. It was expected that I would be in the examination room. I was sitting near the doctor and had a good view of everything. I was expecting the jelly on the belly like you see on TV.

First the doctor inserted a shiny object and checked things out. Then the doctor lubed up a huge probe and shoved it inside her—well, gently placed it inside her. This was the shocking part. My wife made a face but didn't seem to be in pain. Then we saw the images on the screen and a fluttering object. The doctor did more exploring and pointed out that the fluttering was the heart beating. This was the awe part.

—Scot, daughter, fourteen months

***

Welcome to your first gynecological exam (aka Guy-ne visit). The first appointment typically happens around week seven and includes the weight check, urine sample, blood pressure, blood work, medical history, and often, a vaginal ultrasound. Try to be there. And expect it to be a strange experience. I'll be honest: I never liked watching my wife get probed, touched, and penetrated by another man (her doctor is a man). I know the doctor has to do his job so we can have a healthy baby, but no, I don't enjoy watching another man dig into my wife's business. Learn to tolerate it.

What's different about this first guyne appointment is that not only will you be invited to attend, you will get a front-row seat in the examination room. A seat so close you might see her cervix. (**Note:** If you were planning to snap photos, this is not the appointment to do it.) Walking into the gynecologist's waiting room is like walking into a women's bathroom by mistake—when you enter the room, a part of you will want to turn around.

After waiting in the waiting room (an appropriate name for it), you'll be invited into the exam room. You might see stirrups, instruments (look for a metal bird beak), lube, and a box of condomlike things. As you settle into your seat, your partner will get her blood pressure checked and will be weighed. She might ask you to leave the room during her weight check. Before the doctor arrives, she will likely be instructed to get naked from the waist down. You should stay clothed.

When she starts to get undressed, you might not get turned on like you did the night (or morning) you got her pregnant. It's as if her naked body has been transformed, especially her vagina. It might not give off that familiar vagina vibe you know and love. It will start to look different over the coming months.

At this point of the book, I'd like to introduce you to the birthing vagina (BV). The BV is different than the SV (sex vagina). The SV is what you saw when you got her pregnant. The BV is what you'll see when she pushes out the baby. The BV is still a vagina, but not the one that got you into this situation. Think of the vagina like a superhero. When the baby is born, it will turn on its super powers and stretch and expand. Once the baby is here, it will return to original form. It might be distressing to see the BV at first, but you will learn to separate the BV from the SV over time (more about the split multiple personalities of the vagina later).

When the doctor arrives, one of two things will occur: the doctor will welcome you and acknowledge your presence, or the doctor will ignore you as if you're invisible. The latter can be comforting and disturbing—comforting because we don't want to be noticed, disturbing because we deserve to be acknowledged. If the doctor ignores you, there's nothing wrong with introducing yourself to him or her. Considering

THE BIRTHING VAGINA (BV) VERSUS THE SEX VAGINA (SV): A SPLIT PERSONALITY

The sex vagina is the vagina that gets her pregnant. The birthing vagina is the vagina that gives birth to a baby. The SV will return six to twelve weeks following birth.

you're part of the process, the caregiver should care enough to meet you. Better to do it sooner rather than in the middle of the exam (shaking hands would be awkward).

Once the initial chit-chat concludes, the exam will begin. Legs in stirrups, your pregnant partner is now like a car up on the blocks; the doctor will sit down and check out the mechanics. If you find this image disturbing to read about, it might be more disturbing to see (but doesn't have to be). The doctor might insert a duck-billed object called a spec-ulum (a plastic or metal object used to examine the vagina, cervix, and uterus). Depending on your seat, you might see a whole new side of your partner (really, it's not so bad). If you don't want to see this, sit near your partner's head.

If the doctor performs a vaginal ultrasound, you'll see a long probe covered with a condom. The doctor will lubri-cate the probe and insert it in her. While you're gasping for air and thinking, *What the hell is happening? Wow, that's big!*, she and the doctor will continue chatting it up. She might grimace a bit as the probe enters, but she'll just keep talking away.

Once the probe is in place, you'll get a glimpse inside her uterus on the video monitor (although you'll probably have no idea what is what). The vaginal ultrasound is performed to see if there is a beating heart—or two, three, four, or five beating hearts (dear God, five?). Once a beating heart has been confirmed, your doctor will leave the room, and your partner will clean up and get dressed.

Afterward you'll have a short talk with the doctor and go over important information. You'll discuss prenatal issues, talk about foods and activities to avoid (no smoking or alcohol), address your questions, and reveal the due date (more

OB-GYN WAITING ROOM CHITCHAT

If the due date is only right 5 percent of the time, why not change it to the due week? Or make it a due month? While we have touch screen technology, GPS tracking, and video games that make us jump around like morons in our living rooms, we still can't figure out when a baby will be born.

on this in a sec). If you have questions for the doctor, ask them. You should be able to talk to this doctor about anything and everything on your mind. If you can't ask questions, that's a problem. You and the doctor are two of the only people who have seen your partner naked from the waist down—and that's a bond that can't be broken (until she delivers and there is a roomful of people seeing all of her). You should be able to talk to the doctor.

At some point during the first appointment, you'll find out the magical due date. Don't be so quick to clear your calendar. This due date is 95 percent wrong. That's right, it's totally inaccurate. If you're looking for a guaranteed date, call FedEx (but don't ask FedEx to deliver your baby). The due date is a rough estimate calculated by counting forty weeks from the first day of her last period. The due date can change based on the development of the baby.

WISDOM FROM PATRICK (SIX-TIME EXPECTANT FATHER, 25+ DOCTOR'S VISITS)

Try not to do anything to aggravate or upset your wife. Don't act like a know-it-all—no matter how many pregnancies you've experienced, every time is a new experience. Always be supportive and compassionate—this means doing a whole lot of listening rather than talking. Make sure she knows that what she's saying is important to you. Undivided attention is a key component that is sometimes forgotten due to nervousness. The visual aspect is definitely intimidating. I would compare it to staring directly into the sun. You don't want your eyeballs to catch on fire, but man, isn't sunshine a great thing? No pelvic exams for me. It's uncomfortable enough for her, I would imagine, and privacy far outweighs her need for my presence. (My wife agrees.) Be a friend, hold her hand, and try to be sensitive. Her needs should be more important than your own at this time. I've learned this the hard way. I have made many mistakes; the worst one was being preoccupied with my own feelings and not being very supportive of hers. Pregnancy is stressful enough without hurting her feelings.

THE BOTTOM LINE:

The birthing vagina (BV) is an entirely different vagina than the sex vagina (SV). It takes forty weeks for the SV to become a BV. Following the delivery, it takes approximately eight weeks for the transformation from BV to SV to be completed. Then you will be ready for more sex with the SV until it turns back into a BV.

Tip #10
THE REST OF THE DOCTOR VISITS: Escorting Your Pregnant Partner

THE TIP:
If your partner asks you to come to the prenatal appointments, make an effort to be at the prenatal appointments.

THE STORY:
When I asked him to come with me to the appointments, he wasn't open to the idea. He told me that the prenatal appointments weren't that important for him to go to because all the ob-gyn does is measure my belly and check the heartbeat. His reaction was maddening, because in my eyes, he should be there. It's his baby too. Being there would have helped him gain a better understanding of what I'm going through. All my hormonal changes become very trying for both of us and having him there would have helped. I wish he would have known how much it meant to me.

—Jessica, twenty-one weeks pregnant

Whenever I asked questions, I felt like the doctor was thinking, "Why are you speaking?" I just wanted to understand what was happening. When we went to the vet to have our Chihuahua's teeth cleaned, he talked to us for an hour about the two types of anesthesia they use to attack part of the nervous subsystem. The vet gave us ten thousand times more information than we got from the doctor delivering our child. We were thinking of having the vet deliver the next one.

—Anthony, daughter, three weeks

***

Some men go to all of the appointments. Some don't go to any. Some want to go to all but can't because of other obligations (maybe work?). If you can't go to all of them, make sure you know when the most important ones will take place so you can make the time or find the time to participate. Ask your partner what appointments are MUST BE THERE appointments, and make arrangements to carve out time in the future.

> Our doctor made it extremely easy to ask questions. He always asked me if there was anything on my mind. I think he was asking for my benefit, but also so he could get a sense of how my wife was feeling through my eyes.
>
> —Andy, son, twenty-one months

After the first appointment, she will likely see the doctor once a month from weeks four through twenty-eight of the pregnancy. Then it's every two weeks from weeks twenty-eight to thirty-six. Then it's every week until the kid comes out. (**Note:** Frequency of visits can vary based on your caregiver and your partner's symptoms and risk factors.) Going to the doctor's visits isn't just about being there for her; it's a way for you to stay connected and informed. It's like going to class. Hearing about it and getting the notes isn't the same (and your grade will suffer).

> My boss told me to take as much time as I wanted at doctor's appointments during the pregnancy because it all goes so fast. My wife made appointments in the early morning or late afternoon. This way, I could go before work or leave work early and catch the train.
>
> —Jeff, son, nine months

The big appointments include the first one (when you

get to hear the heartbeat) and the twenty-week ultrasound (when you get to see the baby). If your doctor performs a nuchal translucency screening (NTS) test, which assesses your baby's risk for Down syndrome and other medical conditions, there will be an ultrasound around weeks eleven to thirteen. The other biggies include whichever ones she wants you to attend. (Attending the birth is also a good idea.) There might not be an obvious reason for you to go (in your eyes), but just being there helps her feel supported.

If you do get to go, expect her caregiver to check the progress of the baby and listen to the heartbeat using a Doppler. He or she might measure her belly, put her on the scale, and take her vitals. As the due date gets closer, he'll check her cervix, see where the baby is positioned, and ask her general questions. He'll talk about the tests he's performing. He'll go through her wishes regarding the birth plan (more in Tip #73). He'll answer her questions. And hopefully he'll address your questions.

Pregnant women can be forgetful; if you're there, you can help her remember to ask the questions she may forget. You can also help her remember

> We chose our doctor based on how well she worked with other same-sex couples. Word of mouth is the way to go when picking a doctor. We used a sperm bank and we were not prepared to not get our first choice...you need to be prepared for that.
>
> —*Amy, daughter, five*

PREGNANCY Q & A

QUESTION: What percentage of the doctor's appointments did you attend?

ANSWER: For the first one, 100 percent; for the second one, 50 percent; for the third one, I think I went once and that was when the baby was born.

—Matt, father of three

where she parked. I used to write a list before the appointment as a backup just in case one of us forgot to ask about something. When it comes time for questions during the appointment, you might want to ask your partner if she wants you to leave the room. There might be things she's just not up for mentioning in front of you, like the increased vaginal discharge she's been experiencing—not exactly a turn-on (unless you're into that).

Things to keep in mind:

- The caregiver who examines her might not be the caregiver who delivers the baby. Ours wasn't.
- Suggest having her schedule the *big* appointments first thing in the morning or last thing in the afternoon. Weekends are good too.
- Caregivers can be intimidating. If your caregiver is impatient while answering your questions, say something. Most of them don't realize they're doing anything wrong. Let them know if you have a problem.
- If you can't attend an appointment, ask about it. Get her some flowers or a card, or cook dinner to let her know you wish you could have been there. She'll never be happier you didn't go.

THE BOTTOM LINE:

Being there means being present. Being present means being involved, which will make her more comfortable.

Tip #11
THE ULTRASOUND: Seeing It Is Believing It

THE TIP:

Make sure to attend the ultrasound appointments and make sure you get a good night's sleep the night before.

THE STORY:

My wife and I have chosen not to find out the baby's gender, so when it got to the point in the sonogram where the technician said she was going to find out the gender and put it in the file, I closed my eyes. The room was dark, there was a dull rumble from the air conditioning, and I had not gotten much sleep the night before. When I woke up, my wife was staring daggers at me, and no amount of apologies or loving statements could assuage her (well-deserved) anger. Man, what an asshole I was! Now I make sure that whenever she says the baby is kicking, I run to feel for myself, mostly because I want to feel it kicking but partly because I want her to know I am very much interested in what is happening with our baby.

—*Lou, twenty-six weeks pregnant*

> He's an EMT. Nothing surprised him, but he did tear up during the ultrasound.
>
> —*Nancy, daughter, fifteen months*

***

The ultrasound is a must-see event.

If you can only attend two doctor's visits, make it to the first appointment to hear the heartbeat (you're probably already past this one) and the ultrasound (usually around weeks eighteen to twenty). If your schedule makes attending appointments rough, have her schedule the ultrasound appointment far ahead. If getting time off from work is tough, suggest that she make the appointment first thing in the morning, late in the afternoon, or on the weekend.

How many ultrasounds she will have will depend on your caregiver, your insurance (check your coverage), and how the pregnancy progresses. The norm tends to be two to three (sometimes only one). A high-risk pregnancy will likely result in a higher number of ultrasounds.

We had three ultrasounds during our typical pregnancy. The first was a vaginal ultrasound (long probe). This ultrasound confirmed the pregnancy and showed us the heartbeat. The second ultrasound was at eleven weeks—this was like the one in the movies. Not that they had a full crew filming it—what I mean is that the doctor put the gel on her belly and rubbed a little mouselike instrument over it. This ultrasound was used to measure

> When we went for the eighteen- to twenty-week ultrasound and saw what looked like a little penis pop up, my fiancé gave me a high five and started to do a little dance, saying, "That's my man." When the little boy turned out to be a little girl, and what we had seen turned out to be the umbilical cord, his dance turned into, "Oh well, girls can still be race car drivers."
>
> —*Jessica, twenty-one weeks pregnant*

the thickness of the skinfold behind the neck (part of the nuchal fold scan—see Tip #12). The third ultrasound happened at twenty weeks. This was performed to make sure everything was developing properly. The doctor looked at the heart, neural tubes, arms, legs, fingers, head, brain, GI tract, and (turn away if you don't want to see) the sex. You can find ultrasound images online to give you a sense of what you'll see and what the doctor will measure. As for gender, it might be possible to determine whether you're having a boy or girl at the eleven- to thirteen-week ultrasound, but the eighteen- to twenty-week one

POSSIBLE ULTRASOUND SCHEDULE (MAY VARY, CONSULT YOUR DOCTOR OR CARE PROVIDER)

Seven weeks: confirm pregnancy and count the babies (vaginal ultrasound)

Eleven to thirteen weeks: nuchal fold scan to identify risks of Down syndrome (and chromosomal abnormalities and major congenital heart problems)

Eighteen to twenty weeks: Time to check for any abnormal development

will reveal the sex with a higher probability of accuracy—assuming the kid exposes him- or herself for the camera.

Up until the first ultrasound, the pregnancy might not seem real. I mean, I knew it was real, but seeing that beating heart at the seven-week exam and hearing the heartbeat at the eleven-week ultrasound is *really* real. For me, it marked the beginning of the emotional connection. To see it is to believe it. To believe it is to feel it. At the eleven-week

A/V CLUB TIP FOR DADS

Record the twenty-week ultrasound if possible. You can use your phone (if it has video) and record the images on screen, or bring a video camera. Make sure your cell phone has available memory before the appointment. It sucks to have to delete videos and photos to clear memory during the ultrasound. And make sure to avoid crotch shots and random nipple pics. Especially avoid posting those pics on Twitter, Instagram, Facebook, and Pinterest.

Some offices will record the ultrasound on a DVD or hard drive. Talk to your caregiver in advance and find out if they have something available for you. Also check with the ultrasound tech to make sure it's cool to record.

ultrasound, we not only saw it, but we also heard it. At twenty weeks, the baby looks like a little person. We saw it sucking its thumb and rolling around in the uterus.

THE BOTTOM LINE:

Bring a camera. Get ready to see your kid for the first time.

Tip #12
PRENATAL TESTING: They Want Her Bodily Fluids, Not Yours (Yet)

THE TIP:
Get tested for genetic disorders. Check with your insurance—sometimes there are programs that can help with the cost.

THE STORY:
Before we got pregnant, my doctor recommended that we do some genetic testing. We are Jewish and therefore have increased odds of being carriers of several genetic disorders like Gaucher's disease, Tay-Sachs disease, cystic fibrosis, and others. I had blood drawn after my annual checkup and was shocked when I was later told that I tested positive for a rare mutation of the Tay-Sachs gene. This meant my husband had to get tested too. If he had tested positive, there was a 25 percent chance the baby could have it and a 50 percent chance the baby would be a carrier. If we both had been carriers, we could still have gotten pregnant, but we would have had to test the baby via amniocentesis or CVS testing. It turned out that he wasn't a carrier, and I'm so grateful we didn't have to go through any of that. The only hassle throughout this whole process was my insurance—arghhhh! They didn't cover the tests at first. It was only after thirty calls and hours of getting bounced around to different people (I'm not exaggerating) that a helpful rep was able to "suggest" that my doctor code it differently; they then covered the claim! We couldn't get them to cover my husband's test because the insurance said that his tests were experimental. He was able to save a

couple hundred dollars by paying in advance and doing it at a hospital that was part of a community-based group for genetic testing.

—Erin, daughter, twenty months, fourteen weeks pregnant

***

When I wrote the first edition, I was hoping that genetic testing would be more mainstream. Unfortunately, it's still not as easy and affordable as it should be.

Genetic testing is a relatively new tool that can help detect the possibility of certain genetic disorders before birth. Three common tests include those for cystic fibrosis, Tay-Sachs disease, and sickle-cell trait. The tests use blood work from the mom to determine if she is a carrier of the disorders. It's ideal to do the testing before getting pregnant, but because pregnancy isn't always something you can predict, your partner can get tested once you get pregnant.

Consult your doctor or a genetic counselor to determine which tests you need. Even if all the tests come back negative, there is still a small chance of being a carrier, although it's extremely unlikely. If any one of the tests comes back positive, the father will then need to get tested for that particular gene. Most genetic disorders need a gene from the mother and the father to be passed along to the baby. And just because both parents are carriers of a given gene doesn't mean the baby will inherit that disorder. The gene may lie dormant or not be passed along. If both parents are carriers of the abnormal cystic fibrosis (CF) gene, there's a 25 percent chance the child will have symptoms of CF, a 50 percent chance the child will be a carrier (and have no symptoms), and a 25 percent chance the child will not be a carrier and not have the disease (see www.cff.org for more information).

Certain ethnic groups and races have higher risks of being carriers. For example, in the United States, sickle-cell anemia affects about seventy thousand people. It mainly affects African Americans, with the condition occurring in about one out of every five hundred African American births. Hispanic Americans also are affected; the condition occurs in one out of every one thousand to fourteen hundred Hispanic American births. About two million Americans have the sickle-cell trait. About one in twelve African Americans has the sickle-cell trait. Genetic counseling can help identify risk and guide couples.

The most frustrating aspect about genetic testing is that while it's so valuable, insurance companies can be less than accommodating about covering it. It's hard to believe that genetic testing isn't a routine part of the pregnancy process. While most states screen newborns for cystic fibrosis, sickle-cell anemia, and other genetic disorders at birth, they don't require parents to be screened for the genes that can result in a child being born with these disorders. In a perfect world, genetic testing would be accessible, available, and affordable to everyone.

In addition to genetic testing, there are normal screening tests and various diagnostic tests that may be recommended during the pregnancy. Screening tests determine the risk of having a baby with some genetic birth defects. What's nice about screening tests is that they do not pose any risk to the fetus or mother. But screening tests cannot tell you for sure if the baby has a birth defect. Instead,

NEW AND SAFER DOWN SYNDROME TEST AVAILABLE

During my wife's third pregnancy, our doctor opted for the MaterniT21 test. This new blood test is administered to rule out possible genetic complications.

MaterniT21, developed by San Diego-based biotech company Sequenom, can detect fetal DNA in the mother's blood as early as ten weeks into the pregnancy. That DNA reveals whether the fetus has the extra copy of chromosome 21 that causes Down syndrome.

Current prenatal tests, which require a sample of either amniotic fluid or placenta, are more invasive and carry a small risk of fetal injury or miscarriage. Also, if you do opt for this test, find out if it is covered by insurance or if there is a special program available. We got a substantially reduced rate.

(Source: http://abcnews.go.com/blogs/health/2011/10/18/safer-down-syndrome-test-to-hit-market-monday/)

screening tests tell you the odds of your baby having a birth defect based on your age or other factors (i.e., one in fifty thousand chance that the child has…).

Diagnostic tests can give definitive yes or no answers about whether your baby has a particular problem, but unlike screening tests, they are usually invasive or come with a risk of miscarriage. Amniocentesis and chorionic villus sampling (CVS) are the two most commonly used, and both tests are more than 99 percent accurate for determining the presence of these problems; the only negative is that the risk of miscarriage from an amniocentesis or CVS is one in two hundred. When undergoing genetic testing, make sure you check with your insurance provider. Testing can be extremely expensive if not covered.

SCREENING TESTS

Some screening and diagnostic tests during pregnancy include:

- *Targeted ultrasound*: the best time to receive this test is between eighteen and twenty weeks of pregnancy. Most major problems with the way your baby might be formed can be seen at this time. But some problems like clubbed feet and heart defects can be missed on ultrasound. Your doctor also will be able to see if your baby has any neural tube defects, such as spina bifida. This test is not the most accurate for finding out whether your baby has Down syndrome. Only one in three babies with Down syndrome have an abnormal second-trimester ultrasound. In most cases, your doctor can find out the sex of your baby through ultrasound.
- *Maternal serum marker screening test*: this blood test can be called by many different names including multiple marker screening test, triple test, quad screen, and others. This test is usually given between fifteen and twenty weeks of pregnancy. It checks for birth defects such

HELPFUL GENETIC DISORDER RESOURCES

National Library of Medicine's Genetic Home Reference site: http://ghr.nlm.nih.gov

Chicago Center for Jewish Genetic Disorders: www.jewishgenetics.org

(See resources on page 469.)

as Down syndrome (trisomy 18) or open neural tube defects.

- *Nuchal translucency screening (NTS) or nuchal fold scan*: this new type of screening can be done between eleven and fourteen weeks of pregnancy. It uses an ultrasound and blood test to calculate the risk of some birth defects. Doctors use the ultrasound exam to check the thickness of the back of the fetus's neck. They also test the blood for levels of a pregnancy-associated plasma protein and a hormone called human chorionic gonadotropin (hCG). Doctors use this information to tell if the fetus has a normal or greater-than-normal chance of having some birth defects. (**Note:** NTS is not yet widely used. If you are interested in NTS, talk to your doctor. If she is unable to do the test, she can refer you to someone who can. You should also call your insurance company to find out if they cover the cost of this procedure.)

- *Glucose screening test*: the test is administered around weeks twenty-four to twenty-eight to detect gestational diabetes. The patient consumes a drink containing glucose (a form of sugar). If the test shows high blood sugar levels, the woman will need to take a diagnostic test to find out if she has gestational diabetes.

(Source: www.womenshealth.gov/pregnancy/you-are-pregnant/prenatal-care-tests.html)

DIAGNOSTIC TESTS

- *Amniocentesis*: this test is performed in pregnancies of at least sixteen weeks. It involves inserting a thin needle through the abdomen, into the uterus, and into the amniotic sac to take out a small amount of amniotic fluid for testing. The cells from the fluid are grown in a lab to look for problems with chromosomes. About one in two hundred women have a miscarriage as a result of this test.
- *Chorionic villus sampling (CVS)*: this test is performed between weeks ten and twelve of pregnancy. The doctor inserts a needle through the abdomen or inserts a catheter through the cervix in order to reach the placenta. The doctor then takes a sample of cells from the placenta. These cells are sent to a lab to look for problems with the chromosomes. CVS cannot find out whether your baby has open neural tube defects. About one in two hundred women have a miscarriage as a result of this test.

THE BOTTOM LINE:

Know about genetic testing and do it. If insurance won't cover testing, contact your local children's hospital and speak to a genetic counselor. There may be testing programs available in the community or a way to code the test so that your health insurance will provide coverage.

Tip #13
COMPLICATIONS AND SECOND OPINIONS: Read This One Twice

THE TIP:

If there are any questions, GET A SECOND OPINION. What could be more important? If you have access to more brains, use them!

THE STORY:

My wife was on meds from about twenty weeks or so—that's when we found out she had an incompetent cervix. The original doctor we were with wanted to put her on bed rest from that point on, so we went for a second opinion. This guy was a specialist and awesome. He juggled drugs and also put in a support instrument. My wife was being monitored from home for about three months. She wore a monitor, like the one they put on her at the hospital to watch the contractions, twice a day for thirty minutes each time. It counted the contractions and then transmitted them over the phone to a monitoring agency. If she had more than a certain number of contractions, they made her do it again. If she still had more than a certain number of contractions, they called the doctor. It was

I wish we had known that we don't have to "obey" the doctor. We are having our child and ultimately have to live with the consequences of our decisions. We should have asked what the risks were for different things that the doctor "decided" we needed to do. We should have spoken up and made more informed decisions.

—*Lesha, sons, seven months and three and a half*

a major pain, but *way* better than her being stuck on bed rest for the entire three months. In the end, our son came three days before the "due date"—they think he was actually a few days late. I'm just so happy we got a second opinion.

—*Adam, son, eight months*

✳✳✳

There is no risk in getting a second opinion.

Complications can happen. Unexpected issues can pop up. Some are manageable; others can cause serious risks to the baby and your partner. Should a complication arise, tests may be needed to make or confirm a diagnosis. Some of these tests can put the pregnancy or your partner at risk. Take amniocentesis or CVS testing—both of these tests can be effective in detecting problems such as Down syndrome, spina bifida, and other complications. But the tests have approximately a one in two hundred risk of resulting in miscarriage. Whether or not to do it, how quickly you need to do it, and who should do it are questions to consider. It might be worth having a caregiver who specializes in a particular procedure perform the test.

Another issue that can come up is bed rest. Factors like having preeclampsia, carrying multiples, or having an incompetent cervix are a few risks that can result in preterm labor. One way to reduce the risk of preterm labor is to be put on bed rest. It can be for days, weeks, or months. Some bed rest can be completely restrictive (only get out of bed to shower and pee). No matter what kind of bed rest, with her in bed, you'll have to be the one in charge of making sure everything is ready for baby.

The tip and story in this section are a perfect example of why it's important to get a second opinion. If your caregiver offers a suggestion that will dramatically impact the pregnancy or your partner's health, consider getting a second opinion. I know this might seem simple, but pregnancy is emotional, and a lot of women have long relationships with their caregivers. Therefore, suggesting a second opinion might be too sensitive. It's as if you don't trust your caregiver. When facing the unknown, it's comforting to have someone you can trust. And trusting someone can mean not questioning his or her judgment and creating a possible conflict. On top of this, some caregivers have strong personalities and will make you feel crazy for questioning them. Whereas in other medical situations, we get a second opinion when making difficult medical decisions, during pregnancy it's not always as easy for us to do.

But your comfort level and your partner's comfort level are more important than your caregiver's ego. You and your partner need to be completely sure that what you're doing is the right thing. If a pregnancy becomes complicated, there's *nothing* wrong with consulting a caregiver who has managed similar pregnancies. Some caregivers are more familiar with certain complications and conditions. If your caregiver feels threatened, he's not someone who is being loyal to you.

As the nonchildbearing partner, suggesting a second

opinion might not be well received. If you haven't been to many doctor's appointments, it might be less welcome. From her perspective, the last thing she needs is you questioning her doctor's opinion—the doctor she trusts because she's been seeing her since she was sixteen years old, the same person her mom, sisters, and best girlfriends have been seeing. If that's the case, read this tip to her. This isn't about loyalty; it's about reinforcing what the care provider says and making a well-informed decision as a couple. The worst thing that will happen is that you'll realize you already have the best care anyone could ever want.

THE BOTTOM LINE:

A caregiver threatened by a second opinion is a poor caregiver.

COMMON COMPLICATIONS:

Gestational diabetes is a form of diabetes that usually occurs in the second half of pregnancy.
SYMPTOMS: extreme thirst, hunger, or fatigue (but usually no symptoms). Also, a blood sugar value of 140 mg/DL or greater on a diabetes test.
DIAGNOSIS: the oral glucose tolerance test.
TREATMENT: most women can control their blood sugar levels with diet and exercise. Some women with gestational diabetes or women who had diabetes before pregnancy need insulin shots to keep blood sugar levels under control.

Hyperemesis gravidarum (HG) is severe nausea in

the first trimester that can cause malnourishment and dehydration in some women. HG keeps pregnant women from drinking enough fluids and eating enough food to stay healthy. Many women with HG lose more than 5 percent of their prepregnancy weight, have nutritional problems, and have problems with the balance of electrolytes in their bodies.

SYMPTOMS: severe constant nausea and/or vomiting several times every day for the first three or four months of pregnancy.

DIAGNOSIS: if you think your partner might be vomiting excessively, call the doctor, who will check to see if she's dehydrated, which can be dangerous for her and the baby.

TREATMENT: many women with HG have to be hospitalized so they can be given fluids and nutrients through an IV. Usually, women with HG begin to feel better by the twentieth week of pregnancy. But some women vomit and feel nauseated throughout all three trimesters.

Urinary tract infection left untreated can spread to the kidneys. This can cause premature, or early, labor.

SYMPTOMS: pain or burning when urinating; pain in lower pelvis, lower back, stomach, or side; shaking, chills, fever, sweats, nausea, vomiting; frequent or uncontrollable urge to urinate; strong-smelling urine; change in the amount of urine; blood or pus in the urine; pain during sex.

DIAGNOSIS: urine test.

TREATMENT: antibiotics, usually three- to

seven-day course of amoxicillin, nitrofurantoin, or cephalosporin.

Placenta previa is a condition in which the placenta (a temporary organ joining mother and fetus) covers part of or the entire cervix. Placenta previa can cause severe bleeding usually at the end of the second trimester or later.

SYMPTOMS: painless vaginal bleeding during the second or third trimester. In many cases, there are no symptoms.

DIAGNOSIS: an ultrasound exam.

TREATMENT: a diagnosis after the twentieth week of pregnancy, but with no bleeding, requires cutting back on activity level and increasing bed rest. If bleeding is heavy, hospitalization is required until mother and baby are stable. If the bleeding stops or is light, continued bed rest is required until baby is ready for delivery. If bleeding doesn't stop or if preterm labor starts, baby will be delivered by C-section.

Preeclampsia is pregnancy-related high blood pressure. It can also be called toxemia. Preeclampsia usually occurs after about thirty weeks of pregnancy.

SYMPTOMS: high blood pressure (usually around 140/90); protein in the urine; swelling of the hands and face; sudden weight gain (one pound or more a day); blurred vision; severe headaches; dizziness; intense stomach pain.

DIAGNOSIS: blood pressure test; urine test; evaluation by a doctor.

TREATMENT: the only cure is delivery, which may not be best for the baby. Labor will probably be induced if condition is mild and woman is near term (thirty-seven to forty weeks of pregnancy). If a woman is not yet ready for labor, her doctor may monitor her and her baby closely. May require bed rest at home or in the hospital, until blood pressure stabilizes or until delivery.

Premature or preterm labor is when a woman goes into labor after twenty weeks but before thirty-seven weeks of pregnancy.

SYMPTOMS: contractions, either painful or painless, any time during pregnancy, that occur more than four times an hour or are less than fifteen minutes apart; menstrual-like cramps that come and go; abdominal cramps with or without diarrhea; dull backache that may radiate around to the abdomen; increase in or change in color of vaginal discharge; constant or intermittent pelvic pressure.

DIAGNOSIS: monitoring of uterine contractions by wearing an elastic belt around the waist that holds a transducer or small pressure-sensitive recorder. Can be worn at the doctor's office, in the hospital, or at home.

TREATMENT: lie down with feet elevated; drink two or three glasses of water or juice. If symptoms do not subside within one hour, contact your doctor. May require medications called tocolytics or magnesium sulfate to stop contractions.

Ectopic pregnancy is a condition where the fertilized egg implants outside the uterus, usually in the fallopian tube.

SYMPTOMS: slight, irregular vaginal bleeding that often is brownish; pain in the lower abdomen, often on one side, and can be followed by severe pelvic pain; shoulder pain; faintness or dizziness; nausea or vomiting.

DIAGNOSIS: blood tests; vaginal or abdominal ultrasound exam (screening that uses high-frequency sound waves to form pictures of the fetus on a computer screen); laparoscopy (surgery to view the abdominal organs directly with a viewing instrument).

TREATMENT: because the embryo of an ectopic pregnancy cannot survive, it is removed surgically, or the woman is treated with an anticancer drug, methotrexate, which dissolves the pregnancy.

Placental abruption is a condition in which the placenta separates from the uterine wall before delivery. This can deprive the fetus of oxygen.

SYMPTOMS: vaginal bleeding during the second half of pregnancy; cramping, abdominal pain, and uterine tenderness.

DIAGNOSIS: an ultrasound exam.

TREATMENT: when the separation is minor, bed rest for a few days usually stops the bleeding. Moderate cases may require complete bed rest. Severe cases (when more than half of the placenta separates) can require immediate medical attention and delivery of the baby.

Mastitis is an infection in the breast that can happen during pregnancy or breastfeeding.

SYMPTOMS: soreness or a lump in the breast accompanied by a fever and/or flulike symptoms; possible nausea and vomiting; yellowish discharge from the nipple; breasts feel warm or hot to the touch; pus or blood in the milk; red streaks near the area. Symptoms could come on severely and suddenly.

DIAGNOSIS: evaluation by a doctor.

TREATMENT: if symptoms are not relieved within twenty-four hours of the following steps, see a healthcare provider (you may need an antibiotic). Relieve soreness by applying heat (heating pad or small hot-water bottle) to the sore area. Massage the area, starting behind the sore spot. Use your fingers in a circular motion and massage toward the nipple. Breastfeed often on the affected side. Rest. Wear a well-fitting supportive bra that is not too tight.

(Source: www.womenshealth.gov/pregnancy/you-are-pregnant/pregnancy-complications.html)

Tip #14
MISCARRIAGE TIP: Skip This One Unless You Need It

Warning: there's just no good reason to read this tip unless it happens to you. I included this in case you need to read about it. Just know that this tip is here and it's available on the next page to check out if you want to read it. If not, skip ahead to the next chapter on page 96.

THE TIP:

Being strong means sharing with her that you're hurting too. Don't hold it inside or it will come out in other places.

THE STORY:

Our first pregnancy went just as planned. Everything went well. During the next pregnancy, we lost the baby at twenty-two weeks. I got pregnant again but lost that next baby at six months.

For a good month, I cried. It was a long process. At first, everyone asked if we were both okay. Then the concern for him subsided and it was all just me. While I had as much time as I needed to grieve the loss, he had to go back to work. His body was at work, but his brain was still trying to deal with this. He spent so much time watching me and being helpful for me that he didn't have an outlet for his feelings. He's deeply personal and has a "never let you see me sweat" attitude. He always wants to be strong for the both of us. His strength during this time in our lives didn't come from bravado—it came from a place of "She's having such a hard time that if I sit here and cry, she will be a mental case. I need to be strong for her."

I cried for months. Meanwhile, I noticed that he started to change. He would snap at other people over things he never snapped about before. He was impatient and not himself. The emotions had to go somewhere—he needed an outlet. What ends up happening in a lot of marriages with a pregnancy loss is that if a couple doesn't communicate, the wife starts thinking the husband doesn't care and that he isn't devastated or upset. He buries his feelings. Then the couple grows apart and the marriage suffers.

Thankfully, we never got to that point. After noticing his short fuse, we talked about his feelings. We cried together. He needed to talk about it, and I needed him to talk about it. Not discussing it doesn't change anything. Talking about it together is what makes it better. And now we have three beautiful children. As time moves forward, this part of our life becomes smaller and smaller, but it's also the part that proved to me that I married the very best man.

—Jami, sons, seven months and six, daughter, twenty-six months

***

Losing a pregnancy is a loss. It hurts. It's painful. It's disappointing. It's scary. It's stressful.

If you're grieving the loss of a pregnancy, the words on this page won't take away the pain. Grieving is a deeply personal process. Take comfort in knowing that there is a community of people who understand and have been there before. Many of these people now have beautiful, healthy, thriving children.

As many as 25 percent of pregnancies end in miscarriage. Most occur in the first trimester. Many end before the pregnancy is detected. Miscarriage is nature's way of ending a pregnancy that wasn't healthy. There's not much anyone can do to keep this from happening. It's a natural part of the pregnancy process. You just don't hear a lot about it because people tend to keep it quiet, but it's extremely common and normal to a large degree.

Should she lose the pregnancy, one common reaction is for your partner to feel guilt and shame—as if she did something wrong. Reinforce that this miscarriage is nature's way of protecting life and ensuring a baby is healthy and able to thrive. This isn't about what she did or didn't do; it's about nature. Blame nature. There's no shame or guilt.

Once the sadness lifts, you'll likely get pregnant again. And plan on having a healthy child. Once enough time passes, this loss will fade to the back of your mind and become a distant memory. This may be hard to believe when the loss is all you can feel and think about, but all the dads I spoke to promise that it will pass.

Another issue that needs to be addressed is the number of couples who lose a child before birth and then lose their relationship. If there's ever a time to talk and have open communication, this is the time. She needs to know that you are feeling some sense of loss. She needs to know you're grieving too. She needs to know that you're connected. Women need you to be there. And not only do they need to see and feel your sadness, but it will help you to get beyond this.

See, as the expectant father, *you* aren't the one people worry about after the miscarriage. It's all about her: "How is *she* doing? How's *she* feeling? How's *she* recovering?" Very few people think to ask about you after the first week or two. Managing your partner's health and emotions, the family's emotions, and your own is a lot to handle. And for a lot of guys, you don't get much time to grieve the loss. You have to go right back to work and continue life as if nothing happened. If you're struggling to move beyond the loss, find a pregnancy forum online and share your thoughts. Lean on others who have been through this. Talk to a grief counselor who specializes in miscarriage.

When it comes to sharing the information with family and friends, do it sooner rather than later. Ask the people you shared the good news with to share the sad news with anyone they've shared with. You want to avoid having someone come up to you or your partner and ask about the baby. If you need guidance, talk to your spiritual leader, the social worker in the hospital, or a professional caregiver who specializes in preterm loss. You don't need to handle this alone, and you shouldn't pretend to be strong and have all the answers. Your feelings are just as important as hers. Reach out and lean on the community that's out there. Visit the discussion forums on www.DadsExpectingToo .com and share your thoughts. Please just know that you are not alone. In fact, there are millions of people who have been there who now have beautiful families. The pain will ease—trust that it will get better.

THE BOTTOM LINE:

Grieve together, feel the loss together, and then, when you're ready, make more babies together.

THE BABY'S DEVELOPMENT

3

This Part Has Pictures

Your Week-by-Week Guide

Welcome, expectant fathers, to the week-by-week guide.

I love this part of the book. The following pages will give you a peek inside your partner's pregnant belly. It will also give you a sense of what your partner is feeling or might be feeling. Each couple's experience will be unique, but this will help give you a general idea of what to expect. If you want to impress your partner, read this section to her in bed before lights out. Not only will it help you stay connected to her and the pregnancy, but it might also get you lucky.

The following pages offer a quick reference guide. I've even included pictures (who doesn't love pictures?). This section includes all forty weeks of pregnancy (yes, more like

Note: I know you're probably beyond week seven, but it's still interesting to look back at your fetus's childhood (and it's a fast read).

ten months). Want updates sent to your cell phone? Sign up for the free weekly tracker by visiting www .DadsExpectingToo.com.

And if you're looking for a more in-depth medical look at pregnancy, check out the *Mayo Clinic Guide to a Healthy Pregnancy* book. Online, you'll find helpful guides at WebMD.com, BabyCenter.com, Parents.com, iVillage.com, and TheBump.com. You can also pick up one of the pregnancy guides in the bathroom or on her nightstand to get more information.

The following pages should give you enough information to impress your partner. For example, when the baby's hearing is fully developed by week twenty-six, you can be like, "Only say nice things to me—the baby can fully hear you this week." That will impress her (or piss her off, turning you into an accidental asshole—see Tip #17).

First Trimester (Weeks One to Twelve)

WEEK 1

She's not *really* pregnant. In fact, the first week of pregnancy is a nonpregnant week. The reason we start counting from this week is because it's just not possible to know the exact date of conception. So, to calculate the due date, the first day of her last period is considered the first day of pregnancy. In a way, all women are fake pregnant from the time of their last period until they ovulate. It's not until the egg gets fertilized by the sperm that she is *really* pregnant.

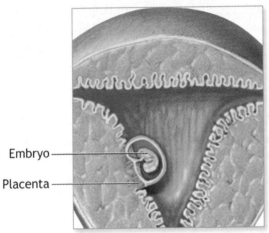

Embryo

Placenta

＊A.D.A.M.

WEEK 2

She's still not *really* pregnant. I know, it sounds like a bunch of crap, but conception doesn't occur until ovulation occurs (that should occur sometime during the second week). That said, this is the week the sperm should fertilize the egg and trigger the beginning of the real pregnancy. When conception happens, two of the forty-six chromosomes that make up your baby's genetic code will meet each other. Because the female egg is always an X chromosome, the male sperm determines the sex. A sperm carrying an X means you have XX, or a girl. A sperm packing a Y means you have XY, or a boy. A sperm carrying a Z means you've discovered a new species of baby.

GRAB ANOTHER BOOK
From the publishers of *Baby Bargains*, make sure to get the latest edition: *Baby 411: Clear Answers & Smart Advice for Your Baby's First Year*, by Denise Fields and Ari Brown, M.D.

Once the egg is fertilized, it will make its way down the fallopian tube and settle into the uterine wall. This is called implantation. Once implantation occurs, the pregnancy hormone begins to release. It's this hormone that will enable your pregnancy test to blink, form an X, form a line, or announce *pregnant* (never seen a talking one).

WEEK 3

Now she's *really* pregnant. Congratulations. No one can tell she's pregnant, but things are happening inside her. It's a 24/7 of things happening. The fertilized egg is rapidly dividing into cells. First two, then four, then eight, then sixteen, then thirty-two, then sixty-four…you get the idea. Eventually all these cells form the blastocyst. The blastocyst is what attaches to the uterine lining (called the endometrium). The area where implantation takes place will become home to the placenta. (This is the organ that acts as the base to the baby and filter from baby to mom.)

3.5 weeks

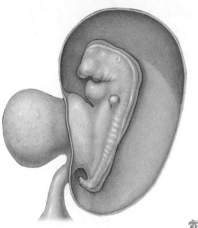

☙ADAM.

WEEK 4

You still may not know you're pregnant. If your partner
has tingling or aching in her breasts (and you're not holding or flicking them), it's the hCG (a pregnancy hormone),
which is also telling her body to stop releasing eggs and
keep the uterine lining from shedding. The switches turning her body into a temple of new life will continue to
flip as she goes into baby-making mode. At this point, the
pregnancy tests with the super-early detection might detect
the pregnancy. Then again, they might not. It's not until
the days following her expected period that the tests will
be conclusive.

WEEK 5

This is the week she misses her period. If getting pregnant isn't a goal, she might not yet realize she's pregnant. As for the baby, things are starting to take form. You're now the proud father of an embryo, and a heart is starting to beat. The embryo continues to make its way into the uterine lining. The neural tube is forming (this becomes the spinal cord and brain). The heart is forming. Also, the placenta is starting to develop. The placenta is an amazing organ that attaches to the uterus and acts as a conduit of nourishment from mom to baby. (Some people will cook it or bury it after the birth.) As for mom, she needs to watch what she eats—no blue cheese, bologna sandwich, or sushi platter with a raw egg dip to celebrate the pregnancy. If you have a cat, don't let her handle the poop. (Congratulations, that's now your job.) The litter can spread toxoplasmosis (a bad, bad thing for pregnant women).

WEEK 6

The brain and nervous system are taking shape. The beginning of the eyes and ear canals are forming. The baby's heart should start beating in regular rhythm at this time. The digestive system, respiratory system, and small buds that will become arms and legs begin to form. All this is happening and the kid is just an eighth of an inch long.

WEEK 7

The big development this week is that facial features are becoming more distinct. There are also hands, digestive organs, and lungs. An umbilical cord is now formed. This will give you something to cut once the baby is born. The mucus plug forms this week. It seals off the uterus from the rest of the world (and that's why sex isn't a problem unless your doctor says otherwise). Beyond the plug, early pregnancy signs may be surfacing (see Chapter 5).

7.5 weeks

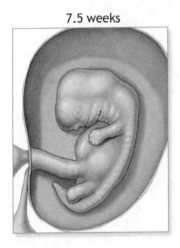

✤ADAM.

WEEK 8

It's bud time—genital bud time. The buds that will form your baby's business are forming. It's still too early to know what you're having, but it's something. There's also pigment in the retina, arms that can flex, longer intestines, and early signs of fingers and toes. Your partner will be feeling pregnant or at least like her pants are tight.

8.5 weeks

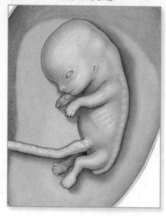

✽ADAM.

WEEK 9

Your kid is now about an inch long and not even a quarter of an ounce. The baby's head is the largest part of the body. Flaps of skin that will soon become eyelids form. Intestines, an anus, and testes or ovaries are also forming. The baby's movement might be visible through an ultrasound, which should show that beating heart (roughly 150 beats per minute).

WEEK 10

Enjoy your embryo because next week, it will graduate and become a fetus. That's right—time really flies. (I remember when you had buds for arms...) At this point, the vital organs are formed. The tail is gone. (Yes, it had what looked like a tail.) Testes, if present, begin producing testosterone.

Fingers and toes begin to separate. The baby looks like a baby. As for your partner, she should have seen her doctor by now. Encourage her to ask the doctor questions. If she can't talk to her doctor, then find a new doctor.

10 weeks

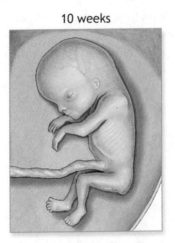

✾A.D.A.M.

WEEK 11

Your fetus is around two inches long. That said, there's a lot packed into that two inches (yes, if you had a dime for every woman who told you that). The placenta is growing at a rapid rate to keep pace with fast growth happening over the coming weeks. Other than that, the ears are moving to their final location and the head keeps getting bigger. (It's half the size of the body.)

WEEK 12

This week, you can raise your glass to little fingernails and toenails forming. Shout hooray for the vocal cords. With new working kidneys, your kid will now be able to pee on him- or herself. Mom's body is pumping more blood than ever. This increased blood flow and hormones cause greater oil gland secretion—this is what may give your partner that pregnancy glow (although if she glows in the dark, she needs medical attention). And with that, she gets a glowing review for her first trimester.

12 weeks

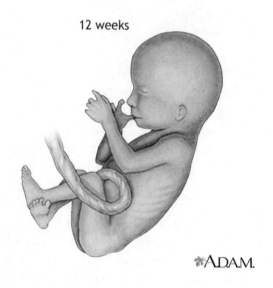

✲A.D.A.M.

WEEK 13

At this point, the placenta is almost fully functional. Think of the placenta as a home base—it's the control panel, and the umbilical cord is the hose that connects the baby to the base. The placenta supplies the baby with oxygen and nutrients, takes care of waste disposal, and produces hormones (progesterone and estrogen) that are vital for pregnancy. At this point in the pregnancy, the eyelids are fused, the vocal cords are forming, and the baby has thumbs that can go in his or her mouth. The face looks like a little person's face. The internal organs are starting to rev up and do their thing.

WEEK 14

Your kid might need a shave about now. But don't worry about these hairs. They're called lanugo and they're said to be soft and colorless (but there's no such thing as colorless). Lanugo will continue growing until about the 26th week, and it will cover the baby's entire body. Lanugo goes away before birth (and it's replaced with vellus hair). The lanugo helps protect the thin skin from the elements. The size of a fourteen-week-old fetus is about one to two ounces (forty-five grams). If you were to stand the baby up, it would be three and a half inches from head to rump.

WEEK 15

For the most part, the body parts and organs are getting strong and growing. The eyes and ears are moving into their final positions. The baby can move its body parts. Soon, the mom will be able to feel something moving. My wife didn't start feeling anything until week nineteen, but it can start sooner or later. The uterus will move higher up above the hip bones to make room for the baby to grow. If you have an ultrasound machine at home (not recommended), by this week you might be able to see if it's a boy or girl—depending on how good you are.

WEEK 16

It's a lot more of the same, but more movement is happening. First-time moms might not feel it yet, but soon the visitor inside will make his or her presence felt. The legs are longer than the arms—prepare for someone to play soccer with mom's internal organs as the baby can kick. Fingernails are present and growing. The baby now weighs around three ounces (the weight of two bags of peanut M&Ms) and measures approximately four or five inches from crown to rump (the length of a package of peanut M&Ms).

16 weeks

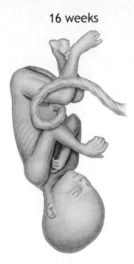

✻A.D.A.M.

WEEK 17

The baby can suck, swallow, and blink. Fat is starting to form. The baby is the size of a grapefruit, a very large orange, or a nice-sized mango. Pick your favorite fruit.

WEEK 18

This is a big week. The baby's ears are in position, and your kid might be able to hear. When you talk, make sure you do it loudly. You're competing against whooshing blood, gas, a heartbeat, and any other noises that might drown out the important things you have to say. The baby is about half a pound or the equivalent of eight ounces of cheddar cheese or Gouda cheese (I love Gouda).

WEEK 19

Speaking of cheese, this is about the time when a white cheesy substance called vernix starts to form. This is more protection for the skin from the fluid in the amniotic sac. This is why your fetus's skin doesn't turn into prunes.

WEEK 20

At the halfway point, your baby weighs in at roughly nine ounces and is about six inches long. The baby is sleeping and waking as if it were a newborn. The uterus is around mom's belly button, which may pop out. The shifting and growing baby will put pressure on mom's lungs, kidneys, stomach, and bladder. But this kid's only half baked.

WEEK 21

The baby continues to develop and organs start practicing. The amniotic fluid carries sugars that can be digested through the baby's intestines. The rapid growth slows down.

WEEK 22

As the brain and nerves develop, the baby becomes aware of new sensations. The baby might move around to test them. If the baby is a boy, the testes begin to descend. If the baby is not a boy, there won't be any testes descending.

WEEK 23

Bones continue to harden, and the baby is just over a pound (or a box of Frosted Flakes). Things are moving in the right direction—like fingers, arms, legs, and toes. If your partner goes into premature labor this week, the baby has a chance of survival with a lot of medical care.

WEEK 24

This is considered the week of viability. Still, a baby born this early wouldn't be going home with mom or dad for several months, assuming it can survive on its own. The lungs continue to develop and prepare for the next phase of life outside the womb. The baby can gain several ounces in muscle this week.

24 weeks

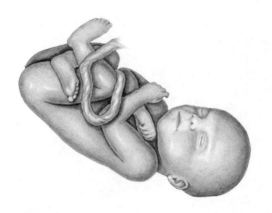

❋A.D.A.M.

WEEK 25

Your partner will feel the baby moving around a lot. The spine is forming. The ears are working and the nostrils begin to open. The uterus is about the size of a soccer ball, and it will get much bigger soon.

WEEK 26

The baby weighs between one and a half and two pounds by now and is approximately nine inches long crown to rump. Brain waves for listening and seeing begin to kick in. At this point, the baby should be able to hear you loud and clear.

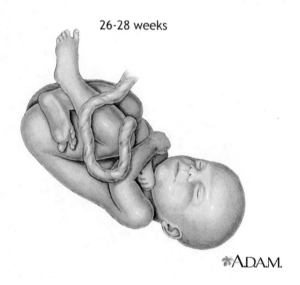

26-28 weeks

ADAM.

WEEK 27

Start saying good-bye to the second trimester. The baby looks similar to how it will look when it's born, but much smaller. But it's growing fast. If the baby were to be born at week twenty-seven, it would have a good shot at survival outside the womb.

WEEK 28

It's now the third trimester. The baby is about two to three pounds (maybe heavier) and ten inches long from crown to rump. The eyes will open, the eyelashes are growing, and there's hair growing on its head. You can talk, sing, or rap for the baby—it can hear you and recognize your voice. The doctor may check to see where the baby's head is resting.

WEEK 29

The baby continues to grow and kick. A normal rate is to feel at least ten kicks an hour. If your partner isn't getting kicked ten times an hour, that's something to discuss with your healthcare provider. They say the baby has a sense of taste by now, so your partner should check with baby to see what he or she wants delivered to the womb and at what time.

WEEK 30

The baby is now about three pounds and getting bigger. It will put on about a half pound a week for the next seven weeks. If your partner thinks the baby might have hiccups, she's right. It's common as the lungs practice breathing. Your pregnant partner might be having a hard time sleeping. Heartburn and constipation might also be a problem for her. Suggest that she sleep on her left side. I'm not just saying that. Research has proven this is the safest side in terms of blood flow to her organs.

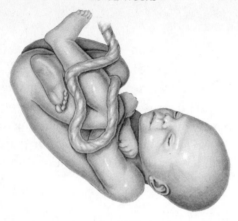

30-32 weeks

✿A.D.A.M.

WEEK 31

The baby continues to grow. The doctor may check the level of amniotic fluid. Too much or too little can be something to investigate. The baby is now peeing several cups of urine a day. The baby's reproductive system is getting in position. The lungs aren't ready to work on their own yet, but they're practicing.

WEEK 32

The baby is about four pounds and eleven and a half inches long crown to rump. The lanugo starts to come off. If the baby was born this week, it would have a very strong chance of survival. Everything should be working. But you still want to keep the baby inside (especially if the nursery is under construction).

WEEK 33

This week, rapid brain growth is happening. Amniotic fluid levels are at their highest. Weight gain continues. Eyes can detect light, so your partner should avoid walking in front of headlights when baby is sleeping.

WEEK 34

More growing—the kid's just getting bigger. While the lanugo is gone, the vernix (the thick coating) gets thicker. You might see this when the baby is born. (They don't show this in the movies.)

WEEK 35

This week, the baby's goal is to gain weight and collect fat. This continued weight gain will make it harder to move. Soon the baby will start to look for larger accommodations.

WEEK 36

At six to six and a half pounds and sixteen to nineteen inches long, the baby might soon drop into the birth canal to prepare for delivery. The doctor will start checking the cervix to see if it's dilated. Refer to the birth section for specifics.

WEEK 37

When this week ends, the baby will be considered full term. Your partner should experience more vaginal discharge as her body prepares for delivery. Don't expect her to show you or tell you about this. The position of the baby is important. The baby's head should be pointed downward by now. A breech baby might mean you have to plan for a C-section.

WEEK 38

This week, the baby could gain as much as an ounce a day. The weight is close to seven pounds. The intestines are accumulating more and more meconium. This is what makes up the first bowel movement (it's like a black tar poop). Your partner might be feeling false labor contractions.

WEEK 39

The baby's getting lower in the birth canal and is almost here. The kid can barely move at this point. Your partner might not be all that steady either; as the kid moves downward, mom's center of gravity can be thrown off. If she works in a circus, no tightrope this week.

WEEK 40

This week, you should meet your kid…or the next week or the next. The average baby is seven and a half pounds and around twenty inches. But none of this is certain. Soon, all hell will break loose. That's covered in the delivery chapter.

4

THE MANY FACES OF THE EXPECTANT FATHER

Inside the Male Mind and Body

Welcome, expectant fathers and your partners. This is the part of the book where you get all the attention. If you're a man, you'll gain insight into the issues you might feel or experience—I'm talking about the things people never tell you but you'll need to know. If you're a woman, this chapter will help you get a look inside the mind of your man. Most women have no idea that their partner is going through changes too.

Tip #15
THE IN-AWE AND HAPPY EXPECTANT FATHER: Words Can't Describe It (But I'll Try)

THE TIP:

It's a feeling like nothing you've ever experienced before.

THE STORY:

Watching each birth was the most moving, happiest, and awe-inspiring moment. It was surreal. It was sensory overload. It wasn't until a few hours after the birth, when my wife and daughter had rested and recovered, that I had a chance to hold my daughter. My wife was sleeping, and we were alone. That was the moment the switch was flipped. It was a feeling I had never experienced before. I was awestruck by the pregnancy, birth, and delivery. The love a father feels for his child blew me away. It's a feeling that never goes away. It happened for the second time when my son was born. This time, it was when he rested on my wife's chest immediately following the birth. The feelings were so intense we decided to do it one more time. Our next child is due in seven weeks. We can't wait.

> —*Me, daughter, seven, son, four, wife thirty-three weeks pregnant*

***

> We had a C-section, and I got to spend time with Jack before Emily did; it's not how I wished it. He opened his eyes and looked at me, and I said, "Hi, Jack." And he looked at me like he knew that was his name. It was the most magical moment.
>
> —*Jeff, son, nine months*

> It's like a Darwinian switch flipped in my brain. I went from reluctant father to head-over-heels committed dad in a heartbeat.
>
> —Eric, daughter, fifteen months

Some men feel a connection during the pregnancy when they first hear the heartbeat. Others feel overcome the moment they see the ultrasound. Some men feel it at birth. Some feel it sometime during the first year of life. For others, it's high school graduation (now, that's a little too long). The feelings will hit you when you least expect it. When it hits you is unpredictable. But it's certain—it will hit.

The experience of being an expectant and first-time dad will leave you in awe. It will excite, exhaust, intimidate, embarrass, intrigue, surprise, scare, shock, and amaze you all at once. The adventure will stir untapped emotions. It will leave you feeling something you've never felt or experienced before.

It's as if there's something programmed into our DNA that's activated during this process. And when the switch is flipped and it happens, the world will change forever. It's an emotional state so powerful and all-consuming that there are no words for it.

Don't worry about not feeling it right away. It *will* happen, but *when* it happens will vary. It could be immediately after the birth, or an hour, a day, a week, or a few months later—but it will happen. It's not something you need to force. No matter the heaviness or happiness of

> I was in awe when I saw the ultrasound of our baby and the heartbeat—that is when I knew it was for real.
>
> —Kevin, eighteen weeks pregnant

the moments leading up to the birth, it will all be worth it. The adrenaline rush of fatherhood is better than any drug—once the initial surge subsides, the feeling lingers forever. It's what bonds us to the baby.

> Enjoy every minute. I would kill to have my girls fall asleep on my chest again or hear the babbles.
>
> —*Moss, daughters*
> *three and five*

From conception to coming home, the whole journey is exhilarating, exhausting, and awe-inspiring. It's something you'll probably want to do again and again. And while you might in fact do it again and again, savor the first time—the first is a once-in-a-lifetime experience. Enjoy the adventure ahead.

THE BOTTOM LINE:
You won't believe what you see, hear, and feel.

Tip #16
THE REJECTED EXPECTANT FATHER: Embracing the URT of Fatherhood

THE TIP:
Sometimes even your smell will make her sick.

THE STORY:
One of my weird pregnancy symptoms was that I could not be touched, kissed, hugged, or held for weeks. I couldn't have him too close either. It got so bad that even the smell of him—you know the smell of a guy—made me queasy.

It wasn't that *he* smelled; it was *his* smell. We didn't kiss for at least a month. This went on for weeks and weeks. I told him that it wasn't anything about him, but I could tell it still bothered him. I apologized whenever I told him not to hug or kiss me, but he looked hurt. After a while, he gave up trying and told me to tell him when he could kiss me again. Once it passed and I was able to smell him, things got better. I don't think he ever quite got it when it was happening. I felt guilty because I could tell I was disappointing him, but I didn't have any control over it.

—*Samantha, son, eleven months*

✳✳✳

Your wife, girlfriend, or partner might not be as into you at times. Don't fight it.

See, there's a force of nature called the Universal Rejection Truth (URT). The URT is an undeniable truth that says not everyone and everything will respond to you the way you want everyone and everything to respond. There are many URTs in life. The URT of dating and relationships says that not everyone you want will want you (thousands will want you, but millions will not). The URT of sales says that not everyone will buy or want what we're selling. The Universal Rejection Truth of being an expectant father says that your partner will not always respond the way you

> It's one thing to have her tell you she's not in the mood; it's another to have her tell you that the idea of having sex with you is so far from her mind that the thought of it makes her want to vomit.
>
> —*Matt, father of two*

ATTENTION, PREGNANT PARTNERS

If you're a woman reading this, it might surprise you that your partner is going through these changes. You might not care because you're going through so much more. Appreciate that this is real. If you can't give him what he wants, remind him that you love him and explain why you can't give it. Never assume he understands. He doesn't.

want her to respond. She might not want to kiss you. She might not want to listen to you. She might not want to have sex with you. She might not understand you or care to understand you at times. As an expectant father, you have a choice. You can either accept the URT or fight the URT.

Fighting the truth means being miserable, unhappy, and resentful. It means getting stuck in a state of rejection denial. Rejection denial is a dark place where you refuse to give your partner permission to react freely to your needs. She will not always give you what you want. Once you can accept this, you can find out why. People in a state of rejection denial get frustrated, upset, or withdrawn. Men in rejection denial take it all personally. They don't understand why they aren't getting what they want. And most of the time, they assume all the wrong things. Embrace the URT. Give her permission to not always give you what you want. When she can't give it to you, find out why. By embracing the URT, you can be a much better listener. Instead of focusing on what you're thinking, you can hear what she's saying—and that will create a deeper a connection.

It's hard when your partner rejects you. She might not always appreciate, include, and desire you in all the same ways. She might spend more time with friends, family, books, or her computer. She might

FEELING REJECTED?
Suggested Reading: *The 5 Love Languages: The Secret to Love That Lasts* by Gary D. Chapman.

not kiss you as frequently or give you as much attention as in the past. Don't think she doesn't love you. It has nothing to do with you. She might not even recognize what she's doing. So much of this for her is about her own self-preservation and her soon-to-be role as new mom.

Once the baby is born, there will be more changes. You'll temporarily go from number two to number three (you moved to number two when she was pregnant). This doesn't mean that she loves you any less; it means that nature has made her a mother, and this role requires her to place her pregnancy and child in priority above you. Acknowledging and embracing the URT makes it much easier to handle it all. Instead of hiding, hating, and resenting her, you can try to understand her. You can listen, communicate, and connect.

Feeling alone at times is normal, natural, and part of the process.

What makes this phase of life even more challenging is that all the changes happening in your life can make you feel more vulnerable and uncomfortable than ever before. Not getting the attention or reaction you're used to getting from your best friend can be discouraging. Some guys look for attention from other women. Some get controlling. Some run away. Some get mean. Some become disconnected. But few expect it, embrace it, and talk about it.

One suggestion to help you get comfortable with the uncomfortable is to have five people in your corner at all times. These people can include friends, family, coworkers, spiritual leaders, a therapist, a doctor, and positive people who have been there and done it. Avoid surrounding yourself with negative people and hot women—that won't help you feel more connected with your partner. Another suggestion is to stay busy doing things that give you pleasure. Plan projects. Take on a new sport. Build something. Grow your business. With people in your corner, things to do, and places to go, you'll always have something to do and people in your life when she's not available.

THE BOTTOM LINE:

She might not want to smell you, kiss you, or touch you. Trust me, it's temporary.

Tip #17
THE ACCIDENTAL ASSHOLE EXPECTANT FATHER: Good Guys Who Make Mistakes

THE TIP:

Even the most loving and supportive guys can be accidental assholes. Your partner will forgive you eventually. (Diamonds help speed the process.)

THE STORY:

My man was an accidental asshole on two occasions in

> During labor, right before the transition stage (really intense contractions), my husband realized that he had left the car at the curb in front of the hospital and left to move the car! I really missed his presence in the room while he was moving the car.
>
> —Anne, mother of four

a very short span of time. The first incident happened before leaving for the hospital. While my contractions were becoming increasingly more painful and regular, he decided that the best thing to do would be to TiVo the Bears game so he wouldn't miss anything. Meanwhile, I was hunched over the kitchen counter and yelling at him to leave the house. By the time we got to the hospital, I was already at four centimeters. Once we arrived and settled into our room, he did it again. We were told during our Lamaze classes that our husbands needed to be sure to eat while we are in labor, but absolutely *not* in the room. So what did my husband do? The first chance he got, he went down to the cafeteria and got himself a nice hot breakfast of eggs and bacon, which he proceeded to bring back up to the room and sit and eat in front of me because he didn't want me to "be alone." My husband was very supportive, but those weren't his best moments.

—Jenn, daughter, two

***

What's an accidental asshole?

An expectant father of twins had a wife who was due at any minute. He went next door to play poker, got drunk, and fell asleep on his neighbor's couch. His wife didn't know where he went and thought the worst. That is, until he came home in the middle of the night. She was beyond pissed. He explained what happened. The loving guy felt awful. Five years later, she's still pissed. This is an accidental asshole moment.

Accidental assholes are well-intentioned men who try their hardest but make mistakes. It might be something we say, do, don't say, or don't do. For example:

- An expectant father who buys his wife lingerie ten sizes too big after the pregnancy.
- An expectant father who goes to the doctor's appointment and makes jokes about her weight gain.
- An expectant father who cooks dinner and forgets to tell her that the salad has blue cheese crumbles.
- An expectant father who compliments his partner's big boobs and calls them better than her old boobs.
- An expectant father who tells his partner that he's tired and achy every time she tells him *she's* tired and achy.
- An expectant father who tells his partner to suck it up when she's in the midst of morning sickness.
- An expectant father who encourages his wife to avoid pain meds because he once had a cavity filled without Novocain and it wasn't too bad.

> I was flying home from Hawaii with my wife and our three-month-old. Turns out that I packed the formula in the checked luggage and boarded a plane for a nine-hour flight! They had to stop the plane and return to the gate so we could get the formula out of the cargo area.
>
> —*Isaac, father of two*

The secret to being a great expectant father is to embrace

your inner accidental asshole. Admit that you were wrong, apologize, and move on. Defending your accidental asshole moment just makes you a bigger asshole. That can turn you into an intentional asshole. An accidental asshole doesn't mean to upset his partner, and he feels genuine remorse when she gets upset. An intentional asshole purposefully disregards his partner's feelings and doesn't feel any remorse when she gets upset. In fact, upsetting her is often the goal (sick, I know).

While few of us are intentional assholes (upsetting our partners on purpose), we will *all* be accidental assholes at some point. When it happens, don't try to explain it—just apologize and try not to do the same thing again.

THE BOTTOM LINE:

We're all accidental assholes. To deny it would be an asshole move, which would make you an intentional asshole, and that's the worst kind of asshole to be.

Tip #18
THE SCARED EXPECTANT FATHER: The Things Men Think, But Rarely Say Out Loud

THE TIP:
The idea of having a baby can be terrifying.

THE STORY:
We had planned to start trying to knock her up in May of last year. But right before then, I was suddenly struck with cold feet, and I told my wife that I wanted to wait to have

children. I wasn't sure if I even wanted kids at all. I didn't feel ready, and I wasn't prepared to give up my happily selfish lifestyle. The truth was I was terrified. My dickish declaration sent my wife into a crying jag for days. Obviously, I soon saw the light—that no one is ever truly ready. You just have to jump in with both feet. Having a child was the smartest decision I ever made—an exhausting clusterf**k.

> Time at the gym is time for myself and a stress release. I need it, and she understands and supports it. From what I hear, time for myself isn't something I'll have much of once the baby is born.
>
> —*Eric, twenty-eight weeks pregnant*

—*Eric, son, fifteen months*

***

Each pregnancy has scared the crap out of me. Admitting I was scared didn't make me more afraid. It actually helped me. Instead of burying my emotions, I was able to work through my feelings rationally and move beyond them. All men get scared. There will be a moment when you ask yourself, "What the hell am I doing?" Questions will hit you when you least expect it. While driving, eating, sleeping.

- Am I ready to be a father?
- Will I be a good father?
- What if there are medical problems?
- Can we afford this?
- What if something happens to her during delivery?
- What if something happens to the baby?
- What if I pass out or can't be there for her?

- What if the baby doesn't look like me?
- What if my partner can't handle being a mom?
- What if I can't be a good enough husband?
- Why does she keep rejecting me?
- Why do I feel so out of control?
- Why do I feel so scared?
- Why is my partner so distant?
- Why am I so overwhelmed?
- Why am I attracted to other women?
- Why do I feel like I just want to run away?
- Will I be as good of a parent as my parents?
- Will our relationship survive?
- Why didn't anyone tell me about this?

Part of being a first-time dad means allowing yourself to feel and experience all these emotions, ask questions, and know that you're 100 percent normal. Expect to feel reluctant, terrified, unsure, scared, out of control, or whatever else you're feeling. To not feel these things is to be an expectant father in denial.

Big life events will fill your head with big thoughts. If you're sixteen and expecting your first, you have good reason to be terrified. If you're twenty-six, thirty-six, forty-six, fifty-six, sixty-six, seventy-six, eighty-six, ninety-six, or one hundred six (which is kind of old for kids) and expecting your first, you too have good reason. These feelings are what bond us together. It's just that men don't sit around telling each other what scares them, and pregnant women don't necessarily want to hear what scares men. We make jokes to cover up what's really happening. A lot of us are freaking out. Now, the secret is out.

Instead of fighting it, running, or hiding from it with drugs, alcohol, addiction, or other women, allow yourself to feel it all *and* not have the answers. Talk to other guys who have been there and done it. Talk to a therapist or mental health professional. Post a note on www.Facebook.com/DadsExpectingToo. Find activities to release tension (working out is perfect).

My prediction (based on hundreds of interviews for this book) is that the moment you look into your child's eyes, the fear and anxiety will melt away. Yes, it's normal to feel apprehensive, to question yourself, your partner, the future, and to feel overwhelmed at times. But try not to let it freak you out too much.

THE BOTTOM LINE:

Feeling scared and admitting it is a sign of strength—it's being a man.

Having a daughter scared me. I always imagined that I'd have a son. I'd teach him things taught the way my father taught me. I felt like I knew how to be the father of a son because I'm a man. I didn't know what to do with a baby girl—like it's some sort of expensive rare crystal that our wives and mothers worry we will damage or lose. I felt like the sex of the baby would somehow change the entire experience, like somehow I would "naturally" know how to mold a baby boy into a man and would simply fumble and bumble when it comes to raising a daughter. I couldn't have been more wrong. I am her guardian, protector, and teacher and I love spending time with her and seeing her develop. She is an amazing, beautiful child, and I absolutely love having a daughter.

—*Fred, daughter, two, sixteen weeks pregnant*

Tip #19
THE "FIGHTING CHANGE" EXPECTANT FATHER: Life Will Change...but for the Better

THE QUESTION:

How do you prepare for dramatic change when you don't know what the dramatic change is going to be?

THE STORY:

At our age and having been married for five years, our life is set as far as being able to go out to dinner at 8:30, doing what we want, going on vacation every six months—but the realization is starting to hit me. There are a lot of things that scare me. I'm worried about things changing—mostly how we will change as a couple. What if that's all she can talk about? What if she becomes one of those women I see at lunch whose only work is spending the day with the kids? I don't want to be one of those couples who just talks about their kids to each other and when they're out with other people. We've always hated those people. I'm more religious than she is, and I don't want to argue about choices we make for the kids. I think back to all the things my parents did for me. My parents were great—they took us everywhere. What if I'm just selfish? What if I'm not like that? What if being a dad doesn't come naturally? What if I have to force myself to be that way? I'm not around a lot of little kids—I

> There's a thought that birth will magically bring a couple together. But it is a profoundly stressful time that continues long after the baby is born. The solace was that we spent time building our relationship.
>
> —*Todd, father, two months*

don't enjoy being around little kids. Will I learn to like being around kids? I'm not great with that stuff. I've never had an interest. You know what it is? I'm worried because a lot of my friends don't seem happy—they love their kids, but they don't love their relationship after having kids. I love our life.

—*Walter, thirty weeks pregnant*

***

I hate change. I especially hate when something costs $1.03 and I only have two dollar bills.

Most guys don't tell you the positive changes that come with becoming a father. They love to talk about all the things you'll lose or miss—sleep, sex, attention, money, and time to yourself. All the things you gain get lost in the conversation—love, life moments, and all the experiences that come with having someone to love, lead, and watch grow. And really, the things you lose are temporary. You get them back later. Kids will last a lifetime.

Sure, the immediate change can be totally jarring, but you forget once you get beyond it. Expect the first three to six months to be exhausting—but again, it gets better. But you have to trust and know that it will get better. If you want it to get better and plan for it to get better, then it will absolutely get better.

Think about it like this—if life is good without a kid, it will get better with one. The things you fear losing will be

> I've been surprised how much having a kid has changed me. I am a selfish person by nature, but as soon as my daughter was born, it all changed.
>
> —*Moss, daughters three and five*

negligible compared to what you will gain. Of course, parenting will change your dynamics as a couple, but if you've been able to handle problems in the past, you'll be able to work through them in the future.

FIVE THINGS TO HELP WITH THIS TRANSITION:

1. **Plan for life to change (in a good way).** If you're constantly telling yourself the change will suck, you're inviting problems into your life. Plan for life to change for the better and it will.
2. **Don't fight it.** It's like a storm brewing. Start building a stronger foundation with your partner now so you can weather the storm. When the storm clears, life will be better—far better.
3. **Be patient.** Be patient with yourself. Be patient with her. Be patient with the baby. It can take a good year to get comfortable with all the changes.
4. **Help yourself.** Read books, talk to other new dads, speak to a therapist on your own or with your partner, exercise, and find a positive outlet to channel the emotions.
5. **You're not alone.** You are part of a community of millions of men. If it sucked so bad, billions of people wouldn't be doing it again and again. Reach out if you ever need help.

For more insight into "The Change" and putting together an "Action Plan" to help anticipate, embrace, and manage the changes ahead, flip ahead to Tip #92.

THE BOTTOM LINE:
Life will change, BUT for the better.

Tip #20
THE EDUCATED EXPECTANT FATHER: Enjoy This Book in the Bathroom

THE TIP:
Bathroom reading can keep you involved.

THE STORY:
The pregnancy wasn't too anxiety-provoking for me. I think what helped is that I did a lot of reading. I read her mom books and a couple of dad books. My wife also had a subscription to *American Baby*, and she would leave the magazines and other reading materials in the bathroom for me. She didn't pressure me to read them, other than leaving them where she knew I'd find them. It took me a while to figure it out, but the magazines all look alike and have the same articles because there are new people constantly going through the same experience. Reading helped keep me involved and up-to-date with the development of the baby. Sometimes, when we talked and she'd bring up something about the development, she'd be surprised and impressed when I expressed some knowledge.

—*Jeff, son, nine months*

***

A man who knows his role, understands birth, and is

educated can be a calming influence. An uneducated expectant father can be a disruptive pain in the ass.

Being an expectant father means facing the unknown and navigating through so many emotionally charged experiences, all of which are new. As we've discussed throughout the book so far, dramatic change can be uncomfortable. Being an educated expectant father means knowing what's coming your way. It's having a baseline of what's normal and to be expected. If you know what's normal and expected, you can alleviate stress rather than elevate it. There have been studies that show having men in the delivery room can increase stress levels for the partner. My take—the studies don't show how calming it can be to have a man in the delivery room who understands the process and is comfortable with it.

For example, if you anticipate that your partner might experience practice contractions (called Braxton Hicks contractions) throughout the pregnancy, the first time she feels a contraction, you can reassure her. Should she want you to have sex with her (a big hypothetical), you don't have to be afraid of poking the baby in the forehead because you'll

> People say that women have a mother's intuition…well, dads have it too. When we had our first child, my husband had never changed a diaper or really ever held a child let alone a newborn baby. I had a C-section and was unable to get up for the first twenty-four hours after the surgery. I watched in awe as my husband fearlessly changed and cared for our newborn son. He said he was nervous before the baby was born, but after watching the nurses toss him around so effortlessly, he knew he wasn't going to break the baby.
> —Jamie, sons, six and two, daughter, four

know that the cervix is sealed tight (plus there's the amniotic sac protecting the baby). Likewise, when your partner sees something strange, feels something new, or experiences something weird, you can calmly help find answers.

By having a baseline of knowledge, you can get comfortable with the uncomfortable. And that means not overreacting, not having to be right all the time, and being a better listener because you're not spending your time worrying and internalizing the experience. Once you have a solid foundation of what's normal, the unknown isn't so intimidating. It just makes this whole thing easier to approach.

Another resource will be the people around you. Find friends who have been there and done it. Ask them questions that are on your mind. Have real conversations with them. Keep them close to you throughout this experience. Also, visit friends with babies. Seeing your childhood friend who is far less responsible than you going through the process will give you confidence that you can do this—because you can.

There are so many resources out there to help you along the way. This book is one. I've also included a number of titles at the back of this book. One in particular is *The Mayo Clinic Guide to a Healthy Pregnancy*. This amazing resource has great information should you want concise medical information. (Of course, you should always be able to talk to your caregiver.) Another resource is the Internet. *Beware*: make sure the information you're reading is from a trusted source. There are a lot of crappy sites out there. My rule is that when reviewing online information, it has to be medically reviewed information. The number-one bookmark for me is MedlinePlus (www.nlm.nih.gov/medlineplus/). Another trusted site is WebMD. At these sites, you'll find links to trusted medical resources and credible sources (but always consult your caregiver). The Internet should never be your final destination to find answers; that's a job for your caregiver.

Other great sources of information are the pregnancy books for women. It's always interesting to see and hear how the information is being delivered to women. *The Girlfriend's Guide to Pregnancy* (by Vicki Iovine) is a classic that can give you a good sense of how women talk to women about these issues. *Belly Laughs: The Naked Truth about Pregnancy and Childbirth* (by Jenny McCarthy) is another. Also, check out her pregnancy magazines. They make for some riveting bathroom reading. Reading a few articles can keep you involved and part of the process. It might even help you get lucky. The more you know, the more comfortable you can get with the uncomfortable.

That said, you can be too educated. If your caregiver isn't concerned about complications, there's little reason to spend too much time reading about them. And really, if you don't like any of the topics in this book because you'd rather not know, just skip them or rip out the pages (actually, ripping out the pages would be a sign of bigger anger issues—reread Tip #18). There's enough to worry about without becoming consumed with what can go wrong. Assume everything will be all right. There's no reason to read about anything other than the good parts (unless you're writing a book about it).

THE BOTTOM LINE:

Become an educated father and get comfortable with the uncomfortable.

THE TIP:

Sometimes she doesn't want answers—she just wants you to answer.

THE STORY:

One day when my son was a couple months old, he was going crazy at home. I was at work, and my wife must have called me three times—over and over again. I can't always answer my phone during work because I'm...working. But she kept calling. When I finally picked up, she was wigging out because the kid was crying. She tells me, "I can't take it anymore. What's his problem? I can't do this!" I told her, "It's gas." And then she starts screaming, "It's NOT gas." I make a suggestion and she yells at me. I can't talk because I'm working. And then it ends up being my fault that he's crying. When I come home at night, he's sleeping and she's back to herself. Everything a guy does is his fault. I'm used to that as a cop—everything is our fault.

—*Mark, son, two and a half, daughter, six months*

***

A man needs his space.

A pregnant woman needs space.

This isn't a bad thing. It gives everyone a chance to step back, reflect, and find clarity.

Here's the problem—with cell phones, texting, Twitter,

Facebook, email, and video chatting, there is no getting away from each other. Technology has made it impossible to be apart. It's easier than ever for our partners to tell us everything that they're feeling, thinking, and experiencing on a second-by-second basis—especially pregnant women and new moms. And it's hard to tell your pregnant partner not to call or text. You can't do it.

She will text, call, and send pictures when she's out on her own doing things to prepare for the baby. Some things you will love to see. But not all. She will text when an idea pops into her head. She will call when she aches. Then, once the baby is born, you'll be able to see and hear the baby crying via text messages, calls, and video chats. Whether you like it or not—you're always on call.

As available as you were before the pregnancy, you need to be even *more* accessible during and after the pregnancy. If you don't answer her call or return a text, it can be interpreted as a lack of support. If you can't talk, explain that you care about her and support her, but you have to do whatever it is that you're doing. The biggest mistake is ignoring her or pretending you're unavailable. If you pick up and she's in the midst of an outburst, patiently listen and wait until the outburst cools. If you do attempt to be helpful and find it's just fanning the fire, stay cool. You can be right and she can be wrong without her knowing you're right and she's wrong (see Tip #46).

> I want to go back to the day when there were no cell phones and I couldn't be reached. Especially on the golf course.
> —Gary, father of three

If you find that you need a break, make sure you have a place in your life where you can find some space. This is where participating in a class (example, martial arts) and having things in your life that require full attention can be helpful. Designate a time in your schedule when you aren't *as* available—going to the gym or taking a class is perfect. You can also find space attending a sporting event, driving, hanging out in windy and noisy places, or traveling to places with no cell phone reception, like underground subways, mountain peaks, or a developing country. There's nothing wrong with giving yourself a short break every now and then. Just don't tell her you can't always be available (bad move).

THE BOTTOM LINE:
You can run out of battery, but you can't hide. Get used it.

Tip #22
THE DEMOTED EXPECTANT FATHER: Standing in the Shadow of Her Belly

THE TIP:
It's like being on the bench when you used to be on the starting line.

THE STORY:
When she was pregnant, I didn't care that she was the center of attention. I'm not one to get jealous of that. After our son was born, it was not what I expected. She breastfed him, so there wasn't much I could do. She would feed him and console him, and I'd stand around. I would try to hold him, but she would tell me there's not much I could do for

> I think my boyfriend was used to being number one in my life. Then he was booted to number two when the baby came, and I really think that was and still is hard for him sometimes.
>
> —Gina, daughter, four months

him. And then, when I did hold him, he would cry and I couldn't do much for him because he wanted to eat. She was taking care of him, and he wanted to be with her. I didn't think this was what fatherhood would be like. I thought I would be a lot more involved. I felt like I was a player waiting on the sidelines—waiting to be called into the game. While I waited, I walked the dog a lot.

> —Phil, sons, one month and two and a half

***

How are you doing? Seriously, I might be the first person to ask you this question.

Once the test turns positive, you drop a rung on the ladder of importance. You move from number one to number two and there's nothing you can do about it. If you're married, it can be similar to what happened during the wedding planning process for many of you. Once she got engaged, the wedding became the number-one priority. After ten months of planning, all you wanted was for things to get back to normal so you could live your life together. The big difference between the love

> I wish I had told my husband, "You will always be the first person in my life, but you may be put in the back of the line a few times. It won't be long before you are in the front of the line again."
>
> —Yasmin, mother of two

train and the baby train is that once the wedding train pulls into the station, we move up to number one again. After she pushes out the baby, we move down another rung to number three (we are behind the baby and our partner).

There are two phases that make up the dad demotion:

- **Phase 1**—Pregnancy Phase
- **Phase 2**—Newborn Phase

During the pregnancy phase, you are no longer the center of your partner's universe. She is focused on taking care of herself, the baby, and figuring out how she'll push a baby out of her vagina. Other people will focus on her, not you. Friends and family will rarely ask about you. "How are you doing?" is a rare occurrence.

Once the baby is born, a mom's maternal instincts take over—and that's when you slip down one more notch on the attention ladder. Most first-time moms don't have a firm grasp on what's happening with the baby or with themselves. It's all new. This is true of most first-time dads too, but moms tend to be the primary caregivers (unless you are a full-time dad reading this). Not knowing what's happening with the baby can be uncomfortable, and uncomfortable people tend to want to be in control. Some moms will want to be in *total* control. What you think and how you feel might not register like it did before. Instead of

> I found the best way to stay involved was to get into setting up the baby's room. I found it fun and therapeutic. It was a way for me to participate and make a contribution.
>
> —*Brian, daughter, twelve months*

letting this new dad demotion deflate you, make it motivate you to stay that much more involved.

Being number three can suck at times—no question about it. But fighting and resenting it can make it suck that much more. It can even make some guys look for attention from the wrong places (see the box about what *not* to do). What expectant fathers need to understand is that being demoted is a natural and temporary part of the process. Don't reach out to the hot neighbor or sexy coworker (bad choices) to find attention and pass the time. After a year or so, the sun will shine and the belly will go away. And so will the shadow you've been standing in.

How to Get Attention When Demoted:

- Attend as many doctor's appointments as possible.
- Share pregnancy books with your partner (and read hers).
- Ask her what you can do to help
- Do things you don't normally do with her (and don't complain)
- Just listen and be there
- Shop with your partner for baby stuff (buy her maternity store gift cards—*don't* guess her size).
- Plan activities. (**Note:** Pregnant women can't ride roller coasters or sky dive.)
- Go on a getaway (a trip is a great way to stay connected).
- Document the pregnancy with photos and video (of her belly).

- Journal your feelings (keep a blog).
- Talk to other guys about things you're feeling.
- Talk to a therapist, health professional, or spiritual leader.
- Go online and be a part of this forum: www.DadsExpecting.com

How Not to Get Attention When Demoted:

- Confide in a hot coworker.
- Confide in a hot neighbor.
- Confide in a hot female friend.
- Confide in strippers (not-hot ones are excluded too).
- Confide in hot online strangers.
- Confide in a hot ex (or any ex who still wants you).

THE BOTTOM LINE:

If you need attention, don't look for it from a stripper (unless your pregnant partner is a stripper).

Tip #23
THE GETTING FAT EXPECTANT FATHER: Proving Your Love, One Nacho at a Time

THE TIP:

She'll get full faster than before. Don't eat what's left on her plate; it will make you fat.

THE STORY:

We wanted to eat out as much as possible before the baby came, thinking that a newborn baby would be noisy and not good at restaurants (not true, by the way). So we'd go out to eat, and my wife would eat part of her meal but become full because her stomach was small. So I'd eat mine and hers, effectively super-sizing every meal! The food was there, and I could not avoid eating it. Portion control was the major issue. I gained a total of twenty pounds during the pregnancy. I felt fat—like the stereotypical overweight dad at little league games. My wife didn't say anything because she always thinks I'm thin. I figured that I would just take it off. Once the baby was born, I went on NutriSystem (Dan Marino's diet). We also realized our gym has a babysitting service, so I got a personal trainer and worked out. It took me a few months to take it off, but it's gone.

—*Jay, daughter, twenty-one months*

✳✳✳

They're not called paternity clothes—they're called fat pants.

I didn't actually give birth to my daughter, but I ate like I was going to. When my wife had our baby, she gained thirty-five pounds and afterward lost twenty of them in one day. I gained fifteen before the delivery and another five pounds after it. I ate during the whole pregnancy and delivery. (I put down my sandwich during the final push.)

There is actually a name for the syndrome that causes expectant fathers to gain weight. It's called couvade syndrome, and there's been clinical research to show that some men also have increased levels of hormones and exhibit similar symptoms as their pregnant partner (but remember, you can never say, "Me too!"). Couvade syndrome can include phantom weight gain (although tight pants are real). It's common to put on five, ten, or twenty pounds. One theory is that a man who exhibits similar symptoms to his partner communicates to her that he's connected and in it for the long haul. (There are hints that our primal relatives share a common approach. In a study cited by *Nature* magazine, male monkeys also gained weight during their counterpart's pregnancy.)

Here's how it happens: when a woman starts craving ice cream, pizza, tater tots, and mac and cheese, a loving partner will join in the action to be supportive. He'll eat it all just so she doesn't feel alone. After joining in for ten months, that supportive partner can get fat—love handles, an extra chin, a bigger pair of pants. Two pounds a month is all it takes.

If you have a history of weight gain or are struggling with weight issues (emotional eating), prepare to gain some weight and struggle. As your family grows, so do your responsibilities (and pants size). Food can be a crutch, and there's going to be a lot of it around you. If your partner watches what you eat (i.e., she tells you not to eat so much crap), don't expect her to keep tabs on you. She'll be too busy watching her own belly to watch yours grow enormous. This means you will have to cut yourself off. Have a plan in place.

Some guys gain their baby weight and keep it on for years. You might be an emotional eater and not even realize it. If you pack it on and can't get it off, get help. I'm a regular at Weight Watchers and have just joined a fitness boot camp. I have friends who are into yoga, marathon running, biking, and martial arts. A perk of losing the weight: it will give you something to do that will give you space and a way to release tension—you're going to need it.

Now, if you happen to lose a lot of weight while your partner is gaining a lot of weight, don't make a big deal about your weight loss. Be quiet. Don't make it a competition. *Never* offer her your old pants. That's one way to guarantee she'll *not* be getting in your pants (see Tip #57: A Guide to Pregnant Sex). Stay active, make working out part of your routine, and start a diet before you need it. Her pregnancy is not a license to eat like a pig.

THE BOTTOM LINE:
Your big man-ass is a sign of your big-man love for her.

Tip #24
THE DO-IT-ALL EXPECTANT FATHER: Making Sure It Gets Done in Time

THE TIP:
Don't leave everything until the last minute. There might not be time to get everything done if your partner ends up on bed rest and you don't have time to rest.

THE STORY:
Having her on bed rest was the worst. She was diagnosed with high blood pressure (preeclampsia) and wasn't able to get out of bed—no preparing meals, nothing other than showering and going to the bathroom. I was in charge of working and getting ready for the baby. I would leave at 7:30 in the morning and come home at 6:30 at night. When

I came home, I had to make sure she got dinner, I had to keep her spirits up, entertain her, and then I had to set up the nursery—cleaning, shopping, getting diapers, bottles, and all that stuff. Her cell phone bill that month had to be about $600 more. She didn't move. It was a mutual appreciation—she was incredible through it all. She was put on bed rest six weeks before her due date, but it turned out to be three weeks because she went into labor early. I couldn't wait for the baby to born. As soon as she delivered, her blood pressure dropped and her weight dropped (she gained ninety pounds). It was like night and day. The couple of days when she was in the hospital were the best. It was the first time in weeks I was able to stop moving.

—*Jason, daughter, four months*

***

You might not have as much time as you think. Remember that the baby's due date is wrong nearly 95 percent of the time. There might also be an unexpected medical surprise that changes what your partner can do and what will be expected of you. Do not plan on her being available during the last month of the pregnancy.

There's always a chance your pregnant partner might need extra rest as the due date approaches, or she may be medically prescribed bed rest by her caregiver. There are different kinds of bed rest (all take place in a bed, but some are more restrictive). Should she get put on bed rest, there's no resting for you, because there's a lot to do. That's probably one reason she's so insistent on getting it all done months before you think it needs to get done. So the best idea is to be prepared. Whenever your due date is, subtract six weeks and make that the date by which *everything* needs to be done. And if you find that your partner can't do what she used to do (because of exhaustion or bed rest), technology and delivery services can do the heavy lifting for you.

Order baby stuff online and have it shipped to your door. Get groceries delivered. Get a cleaning service to come once every two weeks during the final months. When dealing with construction and home improvement projects, *do not plan on her being available to help*. Remember, the due date is about as reliable as the contractor finishing on time. Get everything done early. The worst thing that will happen is that you will have extra time to hang out with your pregnant partner and play with her belly.

THE BOTTOM LINE:

Plan on the kid coming at least four to six weeks early and plan on the contractor being at least four to six months late.

Tip #25
THE PROTECTIVE EXPECTANT FATHER: Watching Out for the Guy in Seat 25D

THE TIP:
If you have to yell at her to stop moving the couch, yell politely.

THE STORY:
We were in the midst of moving when all of a sudden she started lifting things. My wife has always been one to do

it her way—even if her way involves moving sixty-pound boxes and risking her own health or the child's. That's exactly what she did. She would push around the couch to get to the boxes. And she would do it with me right there. She knows that I would do it for her—I'm the one who schleps. I'm sitting there with able hands, and a pregnant woman is moving things. There was nothing I could to do stop her. So I yelled at her in the nicest way a guy can yell. She got mad—I swear it was a polite yell, but she kept lifting. She moved a huge couch to move the sixty-pound boxes. That's how the third trimester started.

—*Chuck, son, two*

✳✳✳

Instincts will kick in. You might feel an overpowering need to protect her. If you're tough, you'll get tougher. If you're not tough, something inside you will awaken. It's nature. You will want to protect her from bad drivers, strangers, random belly rubbers, dangerous food, pain, aches, weirdos, and overeager family and friends who won't leave her alone. Here's how to do it.

FROM RUDE PEOPLE

Not everyone will open doors and give up seats for her (assholes!). Some people will argue with her, upset her, and make her cry. The way to exert control over the things you can't control is to control yourself. When it happens, you'll get pissed. But no one understands. Assume these people don't know she's pregnant or don't care. Give people permission to be stupid and selfish. Complain to me and vent on

Facebook (www.facebook.com/DadsExpectingToo).

FROM BELLY TOUCHING

Women, men, old people, young people, friends, family, coworkers, classmates, and strangers in elevators will reach out to touch it. In addition to getting her a T-shirt that says, "Touch and I Tase," and a custom-made button that says, "Touch yourself, not my belly," encourage her to set boundaries. If someone touches her, she has every right to tell that person she's uncomfortable. The "uncomfortable" word is the least confrontational.

FROM ORDERING HIGH-RISK FOOD

You ask a server if there are raw eggs in the Caesar salad dressing and he says, "Don't think so." And you say, "Do you know or think you know?" And he says, "I'm not sure." Ask him to please find out. People at the dinner table might criticize you or find you annoying, but that's not something you can control.

THE GUY IN SEAT 25D

Once I was boarding a three-hour flight from Chicago to California. I had an aisle seat one row in front of my twenty-week pregnant wife and twenty-two-month-old daughter. When we asked the guy next to them in 25D—also an aisle seat—if he would trade with me, he said "No." His buddy was sitting across from him and he didn't want to move. I can't imagine that he has kids, because no father would separate a man from his family and leave his pregnant wife to take care of a toddler. This is what you call bad karma.

You have every right to ask questions and send back under-cooked food. Instead of attacking the people who give you a hard time when protecting your partner, educate them. If they keep riding you, give yourself the label of the most loving and protective father. If "annoying" is their label, that's not a bad thing to be (see Tip #7 for a refresher).

FROM HERSELF

Pregnant women will do crazy things. They move furniture, do projects that involve breathing in noxious fumes, and generally do too much. Protecting her from herself can be...very sensitive. Whatever happens, remember, it's never cool to yell at a pregnant woman. Even if she's carrying a heavy bookshelf up the stairs, climbing a ladder, or doing something dangerous—hold back. It just makes her yell back or cry. And that turns you into an accidental asshole. If she won't listen, ask her what you can say or do to get her to listen. Have her tell you how to talk to her. If you do lose your temper, apologize. If this takes place after week twenty, also apologize to the baby for yelling at mommy (he can hear ya).

FROM THE ACHES AND PAINS

Giving birth can be painful (so I hear), and there's nothing you can do to stop the pain. You can only help manage it (or ignore it). Helping her with breathing, counting contractions, acting as a strong advocate, finding the best care, communicating her birth plan to the team, being involved, staying informed, and holding her hand throughout the process is the best way to protect her. Just being there is doing so much.

FROM RANDOM VIOLENCE

It's a fact that women are the most vulnerable when pregnant. Remind her to be vigilant and hyper-aware. Get her pepper spray, a whistle, and try to avoid having her do things that will put her in dark parking lots. If you ever hurt or cause her harm, get help. Partners frequently pose the greatest dangers. The risk of domestic violence increases during pregnancy. Some men feel their most unstable and uncomfortable during this time of transition.

FROM FAMILY AND FRIENDS

Be the buffer. Have your partner express herself to them first. Then step in and repeat what she expressed. It's not about you. It's about her. Family and friends might mean well, but sometimes they are too involved and helpful. You need to be the buffer to help her be comfortable, rested, and happy.

THE BOTTOM LINE:

You might want to protect her, but she needs to protect herself.

Tip #26
THE CALM EXPECTANT FATHER: So Cool She Might Think You're Cold

THE TIP:

Sometimes being too calm can cause her to get even more upset.

THE STORY:

I'm probably more calm than my wife wants me to be, but

that's just how I am. I don't panic, because someone needs to stay calm and be in control. During the first pregnancy, she was put on bed rest at thirty weeks, and our son was born a month early. This pregnancy, we've been to the hospital twice and everything has been fine. At around twenty-five weeks, my wife was feeling some discomfort and called the after-hours line. We were sent directly to labor and delivery. They hooked her up to the contraction monitor, but not much was happening. Then, most recently, at about thirty weeks, she felt some contractions and we went to the hospital. This time, the contractions showed up on the monitor, but they weren't cause for concern. Again, they sent us home. When I tell her that everything will be all right, her emotions take over, creating a minor flare. I just don't get scared. I tend to think everything will be OK, but sometimes she doesn't want to hear it. There are some people shitting their pants (pardon my language), but I saw my friends do it and realized it doesn't have to be so difficult. She sometimes feels that I'm disconnected because I'm so calm, but I express my excitement and concern in different ways. When good things are happening, I get excited. When the not-so-good things happen, I need to be mentally in control. So I don't panic.

—*Jon, son, twenty-five months, thirty-one weeks pregnant*

***

There *is* such a thing as a calm expectant father. I'm not one.

If you're a cool and calm expectant dad, your partner might find you annoying and insensitive. Your level of calmness and cool nature could be misinterpreted. The idea that she's freaking out and you've *never* been more relaxed just might not have a calming effect on her. I mean really, as a guy, you have every reason to be calm. It's not like you're the one who is going to have to push a seven-pound baby through your penis.

Being so calm might also make her think you're not concerned. I mean, it's easy for you to be calm because *you* don't have to feel completely out of control. You aren't gaining weight (which you might actually do), getting swollen, getting sick, and having a kid yanked out from between your legs. She may think that, clearly, if you're this calm, you must not be seeing her point of view or understanding what she is feeling.

How could anyone caring be so calm?

The calm expectant father can stay calm, but he needs to make sure to validate her experiences and not negate her. It's the difference between telling her that her aches and pains are nothing and holding her hand and massaging her aches and pains away. It can take work to show her that you're connected. If she feels pain and she's concerned, she'll want you to be concerned. You can be calm and concerned, but she needs to know that you feel her pain.

I agree, if you're going to spend your time and energy worrying, better to spend it on things that are worth worrying about. In most situations, there isn't anything to worry about, and you might have no idea where her emotions are coming from. But if she's worried, let her know that you understand and think that her feelings are valid.

THE BOTTOM LINE:

Remember, it's easier for an expectant father to be calm because men don't have to push a living person through a tiny opening in between our legs.

THE TIP:

Never tell a pregnant woman you're tired too. They don't want to hear it—especially when they're in labor and haven't slept.

THE STORY:

I had insomnia with all three of my pregnancies. I was completely exhausted. My husband would wake up in the morning after a full night's sleep and proceed to tell me how tired he was, as if I was supposed to feel bad for him. To top it off, my first labor was long and hard. It lasted twenty-two hours. He slept sixteen of those twenty-two hours while I was in painful labor. When he woke up, he told me how tired he was after his sixteen-hour nap.

—Joann, daughters, four and two, son, eight months

***

This one took me a while to figure out—women want their own aches and pains.

When your pregnant partner tells you that something bothers her, she wants attention. She wants to be acknowledged. She doesn't want to hear about you.

> I want to feel like I'm the only one in the world who's pregnant. I know other women have been pregnant before, but when I'm feeling something, I want to think I'm the only one.
>
> *—Ellie, thirty-nine weeks pregnant*

> She told me that she was constipated when she was thirty-eight weeks pregnant. I told her I was constipated too. She told me that she didn't give a sh*t.
> —*Matthew, father of two*

When you tell her that you feel the same thing she's feeling, that means *you* want attention and *you* need to be taken care of. And she has too much going on to worry about that.

If your partner is complaining that she has a headache, don't say, "My head hurts too." If your partner is tired, don't tell her how tired you are too. If she says she's nauseous, don't be nauseous too. When she complains about aches and pains, don't talk about your aches and pains (even if you're a professional football player). If she says that she can't sleep at night, don't tell her how you can't sleep either. If she talks about her big belly and stretch marks, you can talk about *your* big belly and stretch marks, but only in an attempt to make fun of yourself. (Weight jokes about her are *never, never, never, never, never* funny—she might laugh, but she'll kick your ass later.)

As much as she loves you, she doesn't want to hear about your ailments. This doesn't mean she doesn't care about you; it just means that she's not interested in hearing about it at that very moment. Chalk it up to the Universal Rejection Truth of being an expectant father (see Tip #16). But don't take it personally.

If you need to complain, preface your complaint by telling her that you know she doesn't want to hear about it, but you wanted her to know so she could understand why it's too hard for you to move the dresser while nesting. It might take cooking dinner and vomiting in the pan for her to realize that you're not feeling well either. Or if you need to complain, call up your mom or your buddies. Tell them that you feel like sh*t and that no one seems to care. You can also post a note online and get it off your mind. I know, man, you're tired. Being an expectant dad is exhausting. Your feet hurt, your head hurts, you're exhausted, you're stressed, you're fat, you have bad skin, you're nervous about the future—I'm here for you, man. I know. I understand. I care. We all care—you just can't tell your pregnant partner about it.

THE BOTTOM LINE:

If you want to complain, see a doctor. Make sure it's not a pregnant doctor.

Tip #28
THE EMOTIONALLY RESERVED EXPECTANT FATHER:
You Gotta Let It Out, Man

THE TIP:

Even the smallest expression of affection can mean so much to her.

THE STORY:

We had just returned from the hospital and his parents came over. I was soooooo tired! The simple fact that they were in the room upset me. I love his parents so much! We get along great, but for some reason, at that moment, I couldn't handle being around them. I went into the bathroom with the excuse that I had to go and just cried! After a few minutes, my husband came in and just hugged me.

He stared into my eyes and told me that everything was going to be okay. He said I was tired and took me upstairs and laid down with me so that I knew everything would be okay. I absolutely love that memory. He was so sweet when he stared into my eyes. He isn't affectionate, so that took a lot for him to treat me that way!

—*Nancy, daughter, fifteen months*

***

Here's how I define the emotionally reserved expectant father: a man who rarely expresses his true feelings in a manner that will reveal a softer side, but loves his wife/girlfriend/partner as much as the most effusive, loving, and expressive men.

This tip isn't about changing anyone; it's about pointing out that if you're an emotionally reserved expectant father, you might need to tell her what you're feeling if you're not good at expressing it. If you're a woman reading this, less expressive does not mean less loving; it just means less likely to express loving feelings as frequently as a pregnant woman might need to see it, hear it, and feel it.

Sure, if you're emotionally reserved, your pregnant partner knows who she's with, but who she is while pregnant and who she was when

> I try to be the typical guy filled with machismo—the type that doesn't cry. After she told me, though, I was instantly filled with all types of emotion that I couldn't help it. I picked her up and gave her a big hug (I'm about a foot taller) and started to tear up a bit while grinning from ear to ear and laughing.
>
> —*Kevin, three months pregnant*

you first met her is different. While she might have been fine with this nonexpressive thing before, pregnancy can change this. She's going to need more—however much it is that you can express.

> I wish he knew how much it means to me for him to *act* excited about the baby. I know he is excited, but it would be nice if he showed it more often.
> —*Amanda, eighteen weeks pregnant*

Whatever you did to show her you loved her before the pregnancy, do it five to ten times more often during the pregnant months. Pregnant women have different needs, and they had no idea how much more affection they would need once they became pregnant. If your style isn't to talk openly about your feelings, then don't say it—just show her. Attending birth classes, getting flowers, buying maternity clothes (or a gift card), attending appointments, enlisting the help of a doula, encouraging her to have a friend participate in the delivery, inviting her family to stay with you during the delivery, giving pregnancy massages, and asking if you can do something around the house (and meaning it) matter. If you have a hard time expressing yourself, check out the book *The Five Love Languages*. I'll mention it in the next tip.

Just make sure she knows you love her and that you're in this together. If you can't say it, find a way to express it. There's no such thing as making your pregnant partner feel too loved—not feeling loved enough is the problem.

THE BOTTOM LINE:

Emotionally reserved doesn't mean less loving. If you can't say it, show it. She needs to feel it.

Tip #29
THE NOT HAPPY EXPECTANT FATHER: When You Know Something's Not Right

THE TIP:

If you sense deep in your gut that there's a problem with your relationship, don't wait for it to get better. Talk about it and attempt to face it together if you want to have a chance of staying together.

THE STORY:

I got married and had kids at a very young age. After we had our daughter, I thought it would get better. When we had our second son, I knew it was too late. I never felt like my feelings were validated. Looking back, I should have been more vocal about my beliefs and feelings. I was always waiting for things to get better, for her to adjust, but it never happened. The blame I put on myself is that I allowed society to dictate what I should be doing instead of listening to my gut. It's like telling a guy who's thirty-five that he's supposed to be married, so he goes out on a date looking to get married as opposed to finding someone he has something in common with. It has to be right. I've realized being a couple is not about forcing a relationship to work, but finding a real relationship that's about mutual respect, love, and comfort. The rest of it falls into place. It would

> Suddenly he discovers a love of community theater that didn't exist prior to my pregnancy! It is such a passionate love that it takes him away from attending Lamaze classes with me! Needless to say, we are divorced now.
> —*Michele, mother of one*

have been helpful, less painful, and less expensive (divorce is costly) to figure this out the first time around.

—*Nick, sons, six months and two and a half*

✳✳✳

Did you know that approximately 10 percent of dads suffer from postpartum depression? I had no idea. It's shocking that no one talks about it (but I'm talking about it). It's real and something you and your partner need to recognize. Most women aren't thinking about it, and most men don't know to think about it. If you find yourself pushing away, pulling back, feeling disconnected, having dangerous thoughts, wanting to run, attack, or hide, get professional help.

If you are having a kid because you think a baby will bring you closer together you're wrong. It doesn't work like that—at least in the long run. It might be an exciting and different angle for a few months, but old problems always come back again. Kids aren't glue. In fact, they just stir the pot and bring more issues to the surface. If you have a history of problems, expect them to bubble up during or after the pregnancy.

It's easy to ignore your problems during pregnancy. And it's easy to continue to hope it will just get better once the baby is born. And then it's easy to get pregnant again. Then you have two kids and the same problems, a cycle that can go on for years. But avoidance just builds resentment. And couples who resent one another split up.

If you weren't happy with your relationship before she got pregnant, plan to do something about it now. If you

MEN AND POSTPARTUM DEPRESSION

According to a study published in the *Journal of Pediatrics*, "Approximately 14 percent of mothers and 10 percent of fathers suffer from moderate or severe postpartum depression resulting in undesirable parenting practices and limited parent-infant interaction." Postpartum depression (PPD) is more than just the "baby blues." These are feelings of deep and prolonged sadness, emptiness, and sense of failure and can include thoughts of suicide. The study continued to mention that depressed fathers are less likely to engage with their children and that pediatricians should screen the parents for symptoms. But considering only a small percentage of men attend doctor's appointments and symptoms surface two to three weeks following delivery, identifying men who need help is that much more challenging. If you think you might be suffering from PPD, contact your local hospital or a postpartum hotline and inquire about referrals for men and treatment programs available in your community. Also check out Postpartum Support International at www.postpartum.net. If you're having thoughts of suicide and you need immediate help, call 911 or the following hotline: (800) SUICIDE. (For more on PPD, see Tip #49.)

feel uncomfortable at times or less important, don't freak out. Get help. In addition to couple's therapy, pick up the book *The 5 Love Languages*. She can read it too (there's even an audiobook). Use this time to understand yourself and your partner better. Find help and support to guide and support both of you.

Once you have a child, you and your partner will always be connected. For that reason alone, it's worth the work to try to fix what's broken. Even if you think it's too late, until you try to fix it, you'll never know. Besides, couples counseling is far less painful and costly than dealing with a separation and divorce.

Couples who want to stay together find a way to stay together.

THE BOTTOM LINE:

Babies don't make problems go away. They just magnify them.

Tip #30
THE TWO FOR THE PRICE OF TWO EXPECTANT FATHER: Twins, Triplets, Quadruplets, Quintuplets...

THE TIP:

Do not fight it. You'll have to devote 90 percent of your time and energy to your family, and nothing could be more difficult or rewarding. It might start off being exhausting, but it will get better.

> Everything was a challenge—having two babies cry at the same time, no sleep. The best advice I have is to make sure the husband gets out of bed as much as his wife does. It should be equal.
>
> —Angela, twin sons, twenty-four months

THE STORY:

We had no idea what was coming. The first thing that popped into my head was complete shock. Then it was, "How are we going to pay for this?" Then it was, "How difficult will it be with two?" We never anticipated this. The pregnancy was hard on my wife. She was sick and on antinausea medication for the first five months. At twenty-nine weeks, she went into premature labor and delivered the babies via C-section. We took one of our daughters home after ten days. The other one came home after four and a half weeks. Having twins was something no one could prepare me for. Basically, for about six months, I got by on four or five hours of sleep and drove 35,000 miles making sales calls. It took a toll on my sex life, work life, and personal life, but I would *not* give it up for anything. Two and a half years later, I look back at what we went through and love it—I would do it all over again. It was the hardest—I went from partying to having no time for myself or my wife, but we came through it. And trust me, it only gets better. My daughters are best friends. They can play with each other and don't need as much attention. We have

> Whatever you and your sleep-deprived wife say to each other between the hours of 11:30 p.m. and 5:30 a.m. is null and void the next day and cannot be used against you in future arguments.
>
> —Doug, daughter, three, son, three

more time to be a couple and to be ourselves. Now, it's the best.

—Kenny, twin daughters, two and a half

***

Congratulations! You're twice as lucky. Two for one sales, buy one get one free, and get the second at half price will have new meaning for you. I have to stop pretending...I would be freaking out if I were you. Two is a lot. It's intense. You can totally handle it, but make sure you have support in place. Find dads who have been there and done it. Drill them. Ask them for as many tips as possible.

Yes, in a couple of years, you will have kids who are best friends. If you're only looking to have two kids, pregnancy will be one and done. It's just that for right now, twins mean twice the work and half the sleep. But I'm told, as hard as it might be, it's so cool to have two little kids once they get over the "I can't do anything for myself" phase.

Carrying multiples means a shorter pregnancy (thirty-seven to thirty-nine weeks is the target), more doctor's visits, additional risks (preterm delivery, gestational diabetes, and high blood pressure are just a few of them), more weight gain (about thirty-five to forty-five pounds is the target), more hormones (and a higher risk of postpartum issues), possible bed rest, possible C-section, and two college tuitions in about eighteen years. (That's not fair, but you have eighteen years.)

Again, the most important piece of advice is to encourage her to have a support network in place before the babies arrive. This includes people who have been there and done

TYPES OF MULTIPLES

- IDENTICAL TWINS: the result of a single fertilized egg dividing into separate halves and continuing to develop into two separate but identical babies. These children are genetically identical.
- FRATERNAL TWINS: the result of two eggs being fertilized by two separate sperm. They are no more alike than any siblings born to the same parents.
- SUPERTWINS: triplets, quadruplets, or quintuplets. Triplets occur in approximately one in seven thousand to eight thousand births, whereas quintuplets are likely to be born only in one in 47 million births.

(Source: kidshealth.org)

it, friends, family, and professionals. Do it sooner rather than later. Once the babies are born (and you don't know when the babies will be born), she's going to be too busy to do much for herself. Start early so you can have a network waiting for you.

Because caring for multiples can be all-consuming, simple things like going out to lunch or going to the mall with the babies is going to be harder for her. She might feel isolated, overwhelmed, or alone. Most women with multiples don't have a lot of people surrounding them who have had multiples

BIRTHING CLASSES

When registering for birthing classes, find out if there's a special class for couples expecting twins. If there isn't a special class, make sure your instructor is aware that you're expecting multiples so he or she can offer you additional instruction and information.

or are pregnant with multiples. When it comes to relating to the experience, having a network of friends (even online friends) can make a difference.

Ask your caregiver to suggest a support group. Also check out the National Organization of Mothers of Twins Clubs, Inc. (NOMOTC). The website offers this description: "NOMOTC is a network of more than 450 local clubs representing over 25,000 individual parents of multiples—twins, triplets, quadruplets, and more. NOMOTC promotes the concept of mutual support for parents of multiples. Opportunities for self-help and emotional support are provided through local and statewide meetings." (Visit NOMOTC at www.nomotc.org.)

When it comes to being a dad of multiples, the physical, emotional, and financial demands can mean working longer and harder than ever before. This is one more reason to enlist as much support as possible—from family, friends, and caregivers (I know, this is getting repetitive, but do it). Investigate enlisting the help of a night nurse to help out for the first few weeks at home. (Babies typically wake up every two and a half hours to feed, but twins aren't always on the same cycle, which means you could be getting very little sleep.) Consider hiring a babysitter once a week—not so that you guys can leave, but so you two can shower and have a few minutes to yourselves. If you're depending on parents to help, ask them for as much time as possible. And about coming home—preterm twins often must stay longer in the hospital after birth before growing strong enough to make the trip home. Once you get home, watch out for signs of postpartum depression in your partner. There's research that points to women who have had multiples as being more vulnerable to PPD.

THE BOTTOM LINE:

Keep your eye out for two-for-one college tuition coupons.

Tip #31
THE ADOPTIVE EXPECTANT FATHER: All the Joy without the Morning Sickness

THE TIP:

Once the waiting part is over, we start to forget about waiting. Like any painful experience, your brain has a wonderful way of forgetting the awfulness. I blame it on sleep deprivation.

> Adoption is an emotional experience. Couples who don't adopt have nine months to get ready. We had twenty-four hours.
> —*Oren, son, seven*

THE STORY:

We've adopted two children. For the first one, we waited seven months until we were matched up with the birth mother. We set up a nursery with the bare essentials

SUGGESTED READING BY AND FOR ADOPTIVE FATHERS

- *The Baby Whisperer Solves All Your Problems: Sleeping, Feeding, and Behavior—Beyond the Basics from Infancy through Toddlerhood* by Tracy Hogg and Melinda Blau
- *Gay Dads: A Celebration of Fatherhood* by David Strah and Susanna Margolis
- *I'm Chocolate, You're Vanilla: Raising Healthy Black and Biracial Children in a Race-Conscious World* by Marguerite Wright

and kept the door closed. Because my wife wasn't going through the physical experience, it was largely a surreal bureaucratic experience that was emotionally wrenching. The waiting process was the worst part. Once our daughter came home, other than the lack of sleep, it was terrific. At that point, my experience wasn't that different from that of a biological father. Having a wife who hasn't given birth is quite nice—this is an advantage of the adoption process. You're not looking after a child with a wife who physically feels like she's been hit by a bus.

—*Andrew, daughters, twenty and thirty-three months*

ANOTHER STORY:

It was a Wednesday, and the social worker called me at work. She says, "So, what are you doing?" I answer, "Just working." She continues, "Anything important today? Because a baby was born on Monday." I asked her, "Have we been chosen? Is it a boy or a girl?" She says, "It's a boy and we want to know, can you get him today?" My husband was in New York and would be there for the next three weeks. I told her, "I can be there." Then I called my husband with the news. That's how we had our second child.

—*Linda, daughter, five, son, two and a half*

***

Welcome, adoptive fathers. I haven't forgotten you.

While expectant dads with partners who carry have forty weeks to get ready, you might have forty hours. You might get the call and have to move fast. There may be no time to process the enormity of the situation. One minute you're a couple, the next you're a family. A lot of the emotions addressed earlier in the book will pop up once the baby comes home.

Adoptive parents have

ADOPTIVE FATHERS AND BIOLOGICAL FATHERS: A SHARED EXPERIENCE

- We share the unpredictable nature of expecting.
- We share the dramatic change our lives undergo.
- We share the exhaustion we feel once the baby is born.
- We share the emotional roller coaster.
- We share wanting to be strong for our partners.
- We share wanting to provide the best care for our children.
- We share the shock and awe of being a father.
- We share the love a father feels for his son or daughter.

unique and emotionally grueling questions and issues that can come up. There's even more lack of control: Will the birth mother choose your family? When will the birth happen? Will she sign over her rights to the adoptive parents once the baby is born? What happens if the baby is born premature? Should you have an open adoption (and meet the mother)? Should you have a closed adoption (where you don't meet)? What will the baby be like? Just like a biological father, until you live it, you don't know it.

Thankfully, you will be supported. With 120,000 parents going through adoption every year (according to the Child Welfare Information Gateway), there are people you can lean on to guide you. But when it comes to the other core issues (see sidebar), I hope this book is helpful in how it touches on the universal themes.

In a way, adoptive parents are even more prepared for what's ahead. You must go through a process to prove you are fit to be a parent. People judge you and approve of your abilities to parent. On the other hand, biological fathers can be completely unfit buffoons and still have a child.

The truth is that none of us know what we're doing, and we all trust that we're fit to be parents, but adoptive fathers have already proven they are capable. And that's a good thing to remember, especially during that first night home when the baby is crying and you're thinking, "Can I do this?" Biological parents have to blindly trust that we can do it. You have an endorsement to prove it.

THE BOTTOM LINE:

Adoptive parents go from zero to Dad in an instant. Expect to be thrilled.

5

THE BODY OF THE PREGNANT WOMAN

Like Puberty All Over Again

It's as if her body has been taken over by another life form—because it has. The next two chapters will help you get an inside look into the mind and body of a pregnant woman. However your partner's body changes, always remember: never touch her breasts without first getting permission. That can be bad—very bad.

Tip #32
THE BODY OF THE PREGNANT WOMAN: Like Puberty All Over Again

THE TIP:

How would I describe how it feels to have a pregnant body? Three words: *out of control.*

THE STORY:

Everything has expanded—my chest (not so terrible), butt, thighs, and of course, belly. Getting dressed in the morning and finding that I've outgrown my favorite clothes is a daily occurrence. Since the third month, there's been a new ache every day. Sometimes it's my lower back, sometimes it's my hip, other times it's a leg cramp. I never know what to expect. The relaxin that my pregnant body is producing makes my joints looser and less stable. I get weird cramps in my pelvic bones when I exercise or move around too much. It's easier to strain different parts of my body, especially when I'm carrying around my two-year-old. My belly button can be seen through my winter coat. It looks like someone drew a line down my stomach with a magic marker. I can't lift and do as much as I could before I got pregnant, which is seriously annoying. Sleeping is no fun at all. I wake up with hip pain and I can only lie on my side. I'm a total stomach sleeper, so I'm tossing and turning all night when I'm not waking up to go pee. I definitely get that this is all for the good of the baby growing in my belly, but please—I'm only in the fifth month. I'm worried about what's going to happen to me over the next four! Don't get me wrong; I love that I'm having another baby. I just like having more control over how I look and feel.

—*Stephanie, daughter, twenty-two months, twenty-two weeks pregnant*

***

It's a hulklike transformation. (She might even turn green the first month.) Her mind and body are in the midst of a second puberty all over again. There's no such thing as being too dramatic when your mind and body are out of control. And this brings me to the one reason why men don't get pregnant. If guys did this, they would be so uncomfortable that they would be totally out of control and kick everyone's asses.

Here's what she might contend with.

HOW DO THEY DO IT?

It's remarkable how women can deal with so much and still find time to work, be a partner, and still be loving. The good news here is that some pregnant women experience very few of the most uncomfortable symptoms, but truthfully, most will experience some of them and additional symptoms not yet recorded in the medical journals. Please send those to me via www .DadsExpectingToo.com.

BURSTING HORMONES

It's like the Fourth of July for months. There's an explosion of estrogen, progesterone, and relaxin pumping. You might think she's just being dramatic, and she might very well be dramatic. (Tell her to stop being dramatic and you'll witness dramatics.) There's a reason for the drama. Her hormones are soaring at levels never before experienced, and her moods might swing. See Tip #42 for more information.

EVER-EXPANDING UTERUS

In order to accommodate the baby's growth, the uterus will grow. As it expands, it will push everything out of the way. Think of walking through a crowded bar on the way to the bathroom. The people in the way are the other organs in the body. She's going to get very uncomfortable. And she'll probably have to go to the bathroom a lot (but not in crowded bars).

The uterus is amazing. It gets a thousand times bigger during pregnancy (bigger than most expectant fathers' stomachs). It goes from a two-ounce balloon that can hold less than a half ounce to two and a half pounds in weight—big enough to hold the baby, the placenta, and about a quart of amniotic fluid. When the baby leaves, the uterus shrinks back to its original size.

INCREASED BLOOD LEVELS

Your partner's blood volume will nearly double during pregnancy (blood levels increase roughly 45 percent). This leads to an increased heart rate and a new look for her with swelling in various places.

EXTREME EXHAUSTION

Pregnant women get tired—more tired than any man can possibly understand. Their bodies are working harder than ever before, pumping more blood than ever before, and carrying more weight than ever before. On top of the physical changes, there's the emotional exhaustion. It will make you tired just reading about it. (More in Tip #39.)

FEROCIOUS HUNGER

Pregnant women need more calories and more food—about three hundred extra calories a day. Some pregnant women go from zero to starving in about one second. If she's hungry, feed her (make sure you move your hands quickly when feeding a pregnant woman). Whatever you do, do not question her hunger or food choices. (See Tip #35.)

MORNING SICKNESS

The surge of hormones during the first trimester can send some women into a constant state of nausea. Some women will have it for months (even the entire pregnancy), and others won't have it all. (See Tip #34.)

TERRIBLE GAS (HERS, NOT YOURS)

Pregnant women get constipated, gassy, and bloated. It can get so bad that they can't control it. Does a pregnant woman get a free pass when passing gas? (More about this one in Tip #36.)

LARGE SENSITIVE BREASTS (HERS, NOT YOURS)

In a matter of days, her breasts will possibly double in size. Don't get too excited. These are not intended to feed your fantasies, just the baby. (See Tip #33.)

VAGINAL DISCHARGE AND HEMORRHOIDS

She's always had discharge, but now she has more of it.

As for hemorrhoids, they're just another one of the gifts that can come with pregnancy. Increased blood volume and pressure on the veins in the rectum make this a common occurrence. (See Tip #37.)

SNORING AND LEG CRAMPS

One reason she might be so exhausted is that it's hard for her to sleep. And with the snoring, leg cramps, and constant trips to the bathroom, it might be hard for you to sleep too. (See Tip #40.)

DEPRESSION AND MENTAL HEALTH ISSUES

Depression can be triggered by all the hormonal changes. It can happen during and after pregnancy. The good news is that it's something that can be treated. (See Tip #49 for more details.)

OTHER FIRST-TRIMESTER ISSUES

- Shortness of breath
- Constipation (be sweet, get her interesting reading material)
- Mild cramping (especially after an orgasm, should you be so lucky to be part of this)
- Excessive saliva (makes for wet kisses)
- Heartburn (makes for restless nights)
- Itchiness (she might need a foot or belly scratch)
- Stretch marks (about half of women will get them)
- Occasional bleeding (never comforting)
- Frequent urination (keep this in mind while planning road trips)

- Headaches (it's not an excuse, it's just incredibly common)
- Body aches, lower back pain, swollen ankles

THE BOTTOM LINE:
It's easier to be a man during pregnancy.

Tip #33
THE BIG-BREASTED PREGNANT WOMAN: You Can Look But Don't Touch (Without Asking)

THE TIP:
Pregnancy boobs are a catch-22 for many men. All of a sudden, you have a real banquet but you aren't allowed to feast.

THE STORY:
They were the untouchable treasure, the forbidden fruit. Hers were extremely large. There was no getting near them because they were always in pain, and in turn, I was always in pain. I would try to get close to them on a daily basis, and she would deny my efforts on a daily basis. I had a name for them, but if I share that name she'll read this and kill me (and I'll never touch any boobs). I never complained or got to the point where my attempts were more than good-natured. I didn't resent her large pregnancy boobs, but I prefer her prepregnancy boobs because I could touch those. I would advise other men to avoid touching and not complain about it. You can't complain, because at the end of

the day, it's not you pushing an eight-pound something out of an orifice. Although, a nice pushing present might help a guy get within arms' reach.

—*Larry, daughter, two and a half*

***

Pregnancy breasts are a big difference. Big. Big. Big.

They tend to take on the personality of the pregnant person attached to them. Pregnant breasts can be unpredictable, sensitive, and irritable at times. They can also be happy, excited, and fun to hang out with. If you're lucky enough to meet them (only with her permission, and never with a handshake),

> Her boobs got huge. She went from a B cup to a D cup. And she didn't yet look pregnant. They were like natural nonsilicone instant breast implants. Those were fun.
>
> —*Eric, son, fourteen months*

you'll discover they are unlike any breasts you've ever met before. They are bigger, more sensitive, and topped with a darker and larger areola (or nipple). And don't be alarmed by an extremely large nipple or two or three (well, three might be alarming).

Most women will go up a cup size (or more). This means a woman with small breasts will have medium to large breasts. This might excite you. But don't get too excited.

A lot of men express a deep appreciation, curiosity, and fascination when it comes to

> If he only knew that those great boobs I had would be tiny again and no longer perky, he would have enjoyed them more…
>
> —*Misti, daughter, two*

their partners' new larger breasts. Whether you're a large breast man or just a large-breasted man, hold back your excitement when you see your pregnant partner's breasts growing larger. A man who gets too excited is a man who risks becoming an accidental asshole. A man who falls over his partner's new big breasts (not literally, but possibly in some cases) might give the impression he's dissatisfied with her regular, everyday breasts. Women are very sensitive to this, and your appreciation can be misunderstood. What a woman doesn't realize is that the majority of men appreciate touching any kind of breast, be it small, medium, large, extra-large, jumbo—

PREGNANCY Q & A

QUESTION: What should a man never do?
ANSWER: Mishandle her tender breasts.
—Suzanne, pregnant
ANSWER: Focus too much on the boobs…they are huge, sore, and become really unsexy during pregnancy!
—Carin, mother of one
ANSWER: Suck on her tender breast.
—Deb, mother of two

QUESTION: What freaked out your man the most?
ANSWER: How giant my breasts were.
—Michele, mother of one

we're just happy to be near one (or two). The excitement of bigger breasts isn't necessarily the size but the experience of something different. It's the cherry on top.

Still, no matter how wonderful, exciting, and interesting you think her new breasts might be, don't let your appreciation get out of control. When you get the urge to say something about her new size several times an hour, instead tell her how much you love her entire pregnant body. If you just want to talk about her new breasts, ask her what she thinks of them. If she tells you that she finds them terrific, feel free to agree. If she tells you that she finds them sore and always in the way, do not offer to massage them and get them out of the way (not sure what that means).

BREAST NOTE

If your partner is nursing (breastfeeding), her breasts will often be sore, tired, and not interested in your attention. Once your baby is done feeding, her breasts will need to rest. Should your partner invite you to hang out with her and her new breasts, be careful if she's nursing. Leakage, spraying, and dripping can occur. Safety goggles might ruin the moment, but be aware of the breast hazards.

THE BOTTOM LINE:

Voluminous, enormous, gigantic, and mountainous pregnancy breasts are for feeding the baby—not your sexual appetite. I know, totally unfair.

Tip #34
THE VOMITING PREGNANT WOMAN: A Sense of Smell that Crime-Sniffing Police Dogs Envy

THE TIP:

Ask what she needs and avoid creating new odors.

THE STORY:

It was like having the flu without the temperature. It would hit me at night. I was throwing up about two to three times on a regular basis. We were living in a one-bedroom apartment, so my husband was always close by, but he gave me my space. I didn't want him on top of me. He would always ask me what I needed. It had to be soup—chicken soup, matzo ball soup, or if it was late, wonton soup or some kind of broth-based soup. I always had a metallic taste in my mouth and didn't like canned soup—it had to be home-made. My sense of smell was magnified a hundred times. Garbage odors and a combination of food smells were the worst. I would walk into a grocery store and want to vomit. I even had smelling hallucinations. When we moved into our new house, I was convinced that I smelled something dead in the kitchen. I'd ask everyone if they smelled it too.

I would point to a place on the ground and they would literally get on their hands and knees to smell whatever it was that was bothering me. Everyone believed me, but no one smelled it. I think it was just a first-trimester thing. Eventually it went away.

—*Lisa, son, twenty months*

***

Up to 70 percent of expectant moms experience nausea and vomiting.

(Source: *Mayo Clinic Guide to a Healthy Pregnancy*)

They call it morning sickness, but it can hit morning, noon, or night. Some women don't get sick at all. Other women get so sick that the vomiting can go on for months (but most will eventually stop getting sick early in the second trimester).

It's hard to watch someone you love go through this gut-wrenching experience. It's a helpless feeling. And after a while, you start to worry about the kid getting tossed around when she tosses her breakfast, lunch, and dinner. Don't spend time worrying. The baby will be fine. Once the nausea passes, it will fade from her memory, but while it's happening, there's not much you can do about it. Just ask her what you can do for her.

When and where it hits is unpredictable. It can be at home during breakfast, in the mall, at dinner, in the middle of an intimate moment in the bedroom, in the car, on a plane, on a train, on a bus, in an elevator, on an escalator, or on a moving walkway at the airport (I love those things). Many times, it's a smell that puts them over the edge.

Why does morning sickness happen? The cause is not completely known, but it's most often thought to be associated with a response to the surge of estrogen and other hormones as well as the relaxing of the stomach muscles, which means food empties more slowly. If it starts at all, it typically begins in the beginning of the first trimester and subsides in the beginning of the second trimester. But it can keep going well into the third trimester (women with multiples, first-time moms, and younger women can have more severe symptoms).

While you can't stop it, there are ways to help:

- Have some crackers or food nearby at all times. Eating something before bedtime and in the morning can help curb the nausea. Keep a little pregnancy box of food next to the bed. It will help her and prevent you from having to get up in the early morning hours to bring her food (unless she always asks you to toast a waffle and you don't want to put a toaster in the bedroom).
- Avoid odors that make her sick (lay off the heavy cologne).
- Don't tell her to suck it up (yes, this has happened). It's normal and it will pass.
- Encourage her to eat smaller and more frequent meals.
- Ginger ale and ginger candies (with real ginger) can help curb the nausea.
- Cook her less greasy foods and more bland foods (don't use the deep fryer).
- Make sure she gets enough rest (this might mean sending her to bed early).
- Talk to your care provider about acupuncture, anti-nausea bracelets, and prenatal vitamins (sometimes they can cause nausea). Also, ask your care provider for advice on when to seek help. Weight loss, vomiting blood or material that looks like ground coffee beans, and no signs of improvement require medical attention.

THE BOTTOM LINE:

Billions of women have vomited billions of times, and billions of these women have had healthy babies.

Tip #35
THE FEELING FAT PREGNANT WOMAN: So Much More of Her to Love

THE TIP:

The more weight she gains, the more often she needs to be reminded of how beautiful she is.

THE STORY:

Unfortunately, I have gained more weight than I wanted to. So far I've gained forty pounds. I was 130 pounds at five-foot-eight. I'm now 170 pounds, and I'm going to gain more. I don't think I'll hit 200 pounds. Getting dressed in the morning is the worst experience; I never know what will fit me.

Some people feel really beautiful when they're pregnant. But I don't feel beautiful; I feel swollen, huge, and unattractive. When I look in the mirror, I recognize my body from the head up but from not from the head down.

The doctor says I'm totally fine. It's particularly hard because all my friends gained twenty-five pounds during their pregnancies. My husband is totally supportive and says that everyone's body is different. He knows it bothers

> If he thought I was too fat, he wouldn't bring me home cookies, right?
>
> —Anonymous

> The first thing he bought me after I had the baby was a jogging stroller to help me lose weight. I told him it hurt my feelings because it made me think that he thought I was fat. He said he honestly knew I'd want to get back into shape and was buying it to please me.
>
> —*Gini, daughter, four months*

me. It probably kills him to see me look in the mirror and get so upset. He's as physically attracted to me and maybe even more so. He tells me I'm more beautiful because I'm carrying his child—even more beautiful than I was before—and I tell him, "You're such a liar." But it helps to hear the words over and over again. There's no doubt that I'll get back to my weight.

—*Allison, seven and a half months pregnant*

✳✳✳

Tell her she doesn't look pregnant from behind. If she looks pregnant from behind, tell her she doesn't look pregnant while sitting at a high table.

Some women find gaining weight liberating. Others find it humiliating. Most women will gain twenty-five to thirty-five pounds (most guys about ten pounds). Some gain more, some less. Avoid monitoring her weight. The end of her first trimester (possibly sooner) will be the end of her normal pants. The end of the second trimester will be the end of seeing her feet. The end of the third trimester will be the end of wearing clothes with a waistline. As her shape disappears, she needs to be reminded of the things she can't see—and that's our job.

As a partner of a woman gaining weight, my very best advice

AND NOW, AN ACCIDENTAL ASSHOLE MOMENT

I was about seven months pregnant and I was looking at myself in the mirror. I started to cry and my husband asked me what was wrong. I replied, "I'm fat and ugly!" His response? "Oh, honey, you're not ugly!"
—Jamie, sons, six and two, daughter, four

is to make her feel beautiful. Some women love their new weight. They find it freeing to no longer have to worry about measuring up to the unattainable body image that society (and men) imposes on them. Others feel fat, ugly, and disgusting. Whichever way she feels, compliment the hell out of her on a regular basis—this way, when she has a bad day and you tell her how beautiful she is, it won't look like you're making it up. She will believe you.

From the point when she grows out of her regular jeans until she has the baby and gets back into them (nine months up and at least nine months down), remind her of how beautiful she is. Find something beautiful to focus on. It can be her smile, eyes, belly, or her courage. If you can't find anything beautiful to compliment her about, then see a therapist. I'm completely serious about this. If you can't find anything beautiful about your pregnant partner, that's not something to ignore.

The following are some things you should *never* say or do and a few things you should *always* say and do:

- NEVER question how much she's eating while she's eating (talk to the doctor if you're concerned).

- NEVER ask her if she "needs" to eat something.
- NEVER ask her, "How can you be hungry? You just ate."
- NEVER joke about how much she eats or what she eats.
- NEVER joke about her weight (even if she jokes at first, it's a trap).
- NEVER buy her clothing that's too big (get her a gift card).
- NEVER use the word *cellulite*.
- NEVER point out the areas where she has put on the most weight.
- NEVER tell her she's catching up to you.
- NEVER point out a problem without having a solution in mind.
- NEVER ask if everyone gains *this* much weight.
- NEVER compare her weight to other pregnant women's weight.
- ALWAYS tell her how beautiful she is.
- ALWAYS tell her how sexy she is.
- ALWAYS answer "No" when asked, "Do I look fat?" (she looks beautiful and pregnant).
- ALWAYS answer "Yes" when asked, "Do you like my body?"
- ALWAYS compliment body parts you love (not just her boobs).
- ALWAYS give her hugs and kisses.
- ALWAYS tell her she does *not* look pregnant from behind.
- ALWAYS ignore stretch marks.

> NEVER point out the food stains on her shirt around her pregnant belly, even if she can't see them...
>
> —*Brian, daughter, one*

If you're worried about her weight, attend a doctor's appointment with her and ask her caregiver about it privately. If she has a history of eating disorders, make sure she mentions this to the caregiver. Hormones and change can trigger old emotions and past eating disorders. In addition to a caregiver, she might need to meet with a nutritionist or therapist to ensure she makes good choices. As a rule, *never* discuss eating concerns while she's eating. If you think she's eating too much or making bad choices, be careful how and when you bring this up.

Most pregnant women will gain two to four pounds per month during the first trimester and three to four pounds per month for the second and third trimesters (twenty-five to thirty-five pounds total). She will need to consume roughly three hundred additional calories a day. If you sense that she's gaining too much weight, talk to the doctor first (this is why it helps to go to the appointments). Do not make food the focus; make it about her physical health and mental health. If you do end up talking to her about it, do *not* bring the subject up while she's eating or naked (both vulnerable times). Discussing it at the wrong time will turn you into an accidental asshole (see Tip #17). Doing it at the right time will make you appear to be a loving and supportive husband.

Another suggestion is to be active as a couple. Plan walks and other low-impact activities. Attend a prenatal yoga class or get her a gift certificate. Change your workout routine to accommodate her.

THE BOTTOM LINE:

Appreciate her new bottom line—it's like being with another woman without the sneaking, guilt, or divorce.

Tip #36
THE FARTING PREGNANT WOMAN: Pregnant Women Get a Pass When Passing Gas

THE TIP:
Make sure the neighbors aren't within earshot.

THE STORY:
At the end of my pregnancy with twins, I was so over it all. I remember leaving for a doctor's appointment, my last follow-up prior to the big day. We were walking (I was shuffling at this point) to the car in our garage, and I don't know what came over me, but I suddenly stopped and just stood there, letting out the biggest fart ever. The sound of it reverberated off the walls of the concrete in the

underground garage. It was so powerful there was an echo that trailed it. My husband and I laughed until we cried, and then all of a sudden, he noticed one of our neighbors had just gotten out of her car.

> Her gas was beyond normal. It would wake me up at three in the morning. Not the sound, the smell.
>
> —*Chase, sons, eight months and two and a half*

She heard the whole thing and was so mortified that when she passed by us, she couldn't even look at us. Mind you, this is someone we spoke with quite often. I really think she wanted to run. When my husband walked by, he said, "If you think it sounds bad, you should smell it."

—*Angela, twin sons, twenty-four months*

***

Yes, women fart.

It might come as a shock to you (and to the woman you love), but all women expel gas. I know—your partner has somehow made you think that she doesn't fart, but she does. And if she has never broken wind in front of you before, take cover—her ass is about to explode.

Many women will become constipated during pregnancy. Along with this constipation comes frequent gas. A lot of pregnant women will constantly break wind. Some of you are used to your partner's frequent flatulence. Others of you are in fart denial (thinking she never expels). Some guys don't mind the gas. Some hate it. Some find it a turn-on (weird, dude).

> Every time I think I feel the baby moving, I fart.
>
> —*Kelli, mother of one, pregnant with number two*

WHY SO GASSY, BABE?

The increased progesterone has a relaxing effect on the gastrointestinal tract. This can lead to constipation, which can lead to gas. A few ways to relieve or manage the gas include drinking more water; eating smaller, more frequent meals; exercising; and asking you to leave the room when she feels the urge coming (you have to leave because she's the pregnant one). Avoid surprising her with meals of cabbage, cauliflower, onion, brussels sprouts, or bean casseroles. These foods are like jet fuel for the colon of a pregnant partner.

Through my personal and professional research, I've discovered that pregnant partners might break wind in bed, in the car, on a train, on a plane, at dinner, at the movies, or on a long road trip. When a pregnant partner breaks wind, what can a man do? Should your pregnant partner get a free pass when passing gas? How to handle her gas can present a serious moral dilemma. It's a question loving and supportive men have struggled with for generations. Options include:

a. Retaliate with one of your own.
b. Humiliate her by shouting, "Baby's got the farties!"
c. Be a hero and take the blame for the public stink bomb by saying, "Excuse me."

Whether it happens on the highway, at dinner, or in the

midst of a sweet goodnight kiss, instead of fighting her gas, exercise kindness and compassion. After all, she can't help it.

At the same time, encourage and promote kind, courteous, and responsible passing of gas. Understand that she might pass a tester. The tester is a test to see if the wind has an offensive odor. Once the offensiveness of the scent has been established, courtesy should be extended to you and everyone else in range. This means opening a window, lighting a match, or spraying the air freshener.

And never retaliate with a fart of your own. Not only is it rude, pregnant women have a strong sense of smell. Retaliation can trigger nausea, which can trigger vomiting. And that's just not fair.

THE BOTTOM LINE:
If she blames it on the dog and you don't have a dog, let it go. That's part of being a loving partner.

Tip #37
THE HEMORRHOIDAL, LEAKY PREGNANT WOMAN: Kind of Like a Leaky Faucet

THE TIP:
If you see something, tell her about it, but wait until the right time. A woman who just gave birth doesn't want to hear, "By the way, you have an inch-wide hemorrhoid bubble hanging out of your ass."

THE STORY:
When she was pushing, a lot of stuff was happening down

there. But I did notice something appearing in her anal area. It was a little smaller than a small raisin. I didn't say anything to her because I didn't know what it was at the time. The female anatomy is a great mystery. When she told me a couple weeks later that she had some discomfort, I didn't connect the dots (no pun intended). She went to the doctor and was diagnosed with a hemorrhoid. When she told me, I said, "Not surprising—let me tell you what happened…"

—*Michael, daughters, two, five, and seven*

***

She might not tell you that pregnant women leak.

A pregnant woman might find herself leaking blood, fluid, urine, mucus, milk, or something else that you've never seen, touched, or smelled before. Women don't volunteer this information, because they want their partners to think they're beautiful and attractive. Leaking isn't hot.

As the pregnancy progresses, you might encounter or hear about an occasional surprise. There's going to be the mucous plug (also known as bloody show). There might be blood from a hemorrhoid. There may be amniotic fluid (if the bag of water should break). There is also urine from incontinence. If nursing, breast milk might drip, spray, or spritz at unexpected times (*do* tell her if wet spots suddenly appear on the upper half of her shirt). During the actual labor and delivery, you might see something that she can't see—things you never wanted to see or thought you would see.

Should you encounter blood or a strange odor at some point, or if you just see something out of the ordinary, say something to her about it. Do not keep it a secret. A woman needs to know.

Knowing how to tell her takes some finesse. Pregnant women want to know that you think they are beautiful, especially when their bodies are out of control. When you see, touch, or smell something, wait a few minutes until the moment has passed (if it freaks you out, wait until you're back under control before explaining what happened). When sharing uncomfortable information, I find the best approach is to sandwich the comment between two compliments. First you say what you love about her, then share what you've seen, smelled, touched, or tasted (yes, it can happen). Once you share it, top it off with something that will remind her that you love her and that you still think she's beautiful.

If you just can't say it, then pull the doctor aside or have someone close to her say it for you. But someone needs to say it.

GETTING TO KNOW HER LEAKAGE

- THE MUCOUS PLUG: Should you spot bloody (brownish or red-tinged) mucous discharge in the third trimester, this is probably the mucous plug (it's what blocks the cervix). Losing her mucous plug usually means her cervix is dilating (opening up) and effacing (becoming thinner and softer). Labor could start right away or may still be days away.
- AMNIOTIC FLUID: The term *water breaking* refers to the amniotic fluid leaking from the amniotic sac (also called *rupture of membranes*). When her water breaks, it can be a trickle or a gush (only about 10 percent of women's water will break naturally).
- URINE: Don't try to make her laugh or tickle her; she will literally pee in her pants. The pressure of the baby on the bladder can make it hard for her to hold urine.
- VAGINAL DISCHARGE: Women will normally have an increase in vaginal discharge during pregnancy—not something you probably want to hear or talk about. If you find that it's odorless or barely has a smell, that's normal. If it's greenish, yellowish, gray, thick, or strong/foul smelling, let her know. This could mean an infection.

THE BOTTOM LINE:

If you see, taste, or touch something that she can't see, taste, or touch...tell her.

Tip #38
THE SPOTTING, CRAMPING PREGNANT WOMAN: Normal and Not Normal Stuff That Might Scare Her (and You)

THE TIP:

She might bleed—don't panic if it happens, but get a hold of your doctor or get her to a hospital to make sure it's nothing.

THE STORY:

She started bleeding late into the pregnancy. She was scared when she told me. She called the doctor, and we were told to go straight to the emergency room. The ride took forever, but we didn't have to wait around. The doctor examined her right away. The placenta was tearing away from the lining of the uterus, which was causing the bleeding. We were lucky that we moved so quickly; it could have been much worse. It was too soon to deliver the baby so she was put on bed rest. Staying in bed kept her stable. She had the baby a month later, about four weeks early. The baby was small, but healthy. That was our scariest moment.

—*Steven, son, three months*

BONUS TIP:

Listen to her body and listen to her.

THE STORY:

Twenty-five weeks into the pregnancy, my wife started feeling pain in her stomach. She said she felt cramping. I told her to sleep it off because we had no problem and no history. Each hour got a little bit worse. For the next five or six hours, she was in pain. Looking back, they were contractions. I was thinking it was ridiculous to go the hospital. It was only twenty-five weeks into the pregnancy. I literally didn't think we

BLEEDING

Up to 25 percent of pregnant women have light vaginal bleeding, or spotting, during the first trimester. In most cases, spotting (light bleeding) is NOT a sign of a problem. But always have her check with her caregiver.

(Source: *Mayo Clinic Guide to a Healthy Pregnancy*)

were having a baby. As we got to the hospital, no one there thought we were having a child either. We thought they were Braxton Hicks contractions. Everything seemed to still be fine. It was about 1:00 a.m., and we expected to be home in a half hour. Then the resident comes in and checks my wife. She reaches her hand up there, and all of a sudden, the resident has a horrified look on her face. She was in shock. She was not expecting to touch a leg. When she reached up there, the baby kicked through. My wife was in labor. She was dilated six centimeters. The next thing I know, I'm like "WHAT THE HELL IS HAPPENING?" The anesthesiologist and neonatologist come in, we sign papers, and they start prepping for surgery, telling us that they are going to have to deliver the baby. Six hours later,

FALSE CONTRACTIONS (BRAXTON HICKS)

The uterus's "practice" contractions can start as early as week twenty-two. One way to tell that they're practice contractions is to have her change her position (from sitting to lying down or from sitting to walking). If the movement slows or stops the contractions, it's most likely false labor. Real contractions will continue and get more intense. Whatever the contractions end up to be, have her call your caregiver to make sure it's not preterm labor.

I was a dad. My daughter weighed one pound, thirteen ounces. She was in the ventilator thirteen hours following her birth. Three months later, we left the NICU and took our daughter home. She is now a healthy two-and-a-half-year-old beautiful girl.

—Dan, daughter, two and a half, son, four months

***

At some point, she's going to turn to you and tell you she's having some pain, bleeding, cramping, or discomfort. And that's going to be the moment your world stops for one very long second—even though it's probably nothing to worry about. The third time around, my heart still skips a beat.

For example, during my wife's first pregnancy, she started getting cramps at sixteen weeks that were so bad, she had to sit on the floor at Target while out shopping. The cramps stopped and returned a couple more times. She called the doctor. He told her to stay off her feet and monitor the cramping. The cramping was either due to a bladder infection or related to her ligaments stretching. Now, I didn't exactly curl up in the fetal position and bite my nails under a blanket of fear, but it was a little scary to think something *could* happen. At least it was at Target (I love Target).

And then there are the days later in the pregnancy. Weird stuff is almost a regular occurrence. Practice contractions can make a first-time mom think she's going into labor. When my wife was at week thirty-eight, she had sixty minutes of contractions. They seemed like real labor as opposed to false labor (see the sidebar to the right), exhibiting all the symptoms of the real deal:

1. They occurred at regular intervals.
2. They lasted at least thirty seconds and got longer in duration.
3. They didn't go away when she changed positions.
4. They were in her lower back and lower abdomen.

I insisted that she was in labor and told her to start packing. I tracked each contraction in a notebook. After an hour, she got tired of counting and fell asleep. Three weeks later, we had the baby (and no, she wasn't in labor for three weeks; they were just Braxton Hicks contractions).

Part of being pregnant means experiencing aches, pains, discomfort, and possibly bleeding. Contractions and cramping will happen at some point. Always call your caregiver if you're concerned. Always call if she experiences the following symptoms:

- Bleeding or leaking fluid from the vagina
- Sudden or severe swelling in the face, hands, or fingers
- Severe or long-lasting headaches
- Discomfort, pain, or cramping in the lower abdomen
- Fever or chills
- Vomiting or persistent nausea
- Discomfort, pain, or burning with urination
- Problems seeing or blurred vision
- Dizziness
- A change in the baby's movement
- Suspecting the baby is moving less than it normally had been after twenty-eight weeks of pregnancy (if you count fewer than ten movements in two hours or less)

When something doesn't feel right, call your caregiver. Don't worry about being annoying. And a reminder: this book is *not* a medical guide. Your caregiver is your guide; always call your caregiver when you suspect a problem. If you want more information to help get comfortable with the uncomfortable, check out the *Mayo Clinic Guide to a Healthy Pregnancy* or consult a trusted website. You can also check out MedlinePlus: www.nlm.nih.gov/medlineplus. It includes a list of resources and publications from respected sources. But again, none of these are substitutes for talking to your caregiver.

THE BOTTOM LINE:
I never knew that bleeding and cramping can be normal. Now you know too.

Tip #39
THE NEVER-SO-TIRED PREGNANT WOMAN: Making Narcoleptics Look Well-Rested

THE TIP:
If a woman says she's tired, help her; don't criticize her.

THE STORY:
I was so exhausted from just being pregnant, and he was supposed to help clean the house. I really needed to take a break. When I told him I was going to lie down, he said, "I don't know where; there's crap everywhere!" I immediately felt guilty about lying down and forced myself to keep going. I remember being in tears because I was so tired and my back hurt. He really didn't understand how tired I was. I should have been more vocal. The second pregnancy, I started to speak up.

—Hannah, son, one, five weeks pregnant

✳✳✳

Flowers and gifts and date nights are nice, but doing the dishes or laundry or making dinner is even more appreciated. Be a partner to your partner, not just a fan club.

—Jon, son, three, thirty-three weeks pregnant

There will be times when your partner says or does something that will make you question whether she's being overdramatic. The best advice is not to say anything. She can be dramatic. It's her right. In fact, I made this mistake so you don't have to. Here's what happened…

HELP HER, AND HELP YOURSELF GET LUCKY

As you'll read in Tip #57: A Guide to Pregnant Sex, cleaning and helping around the house will help her save her energy for later. In the words of one woman, "She has a finite amount of energy. Helping out means she might be able to expend some energy on you."

At the time, my wife was nine weeks into her second pregnancy. We had a conversation on the phone during which it sounded like she could hardly push the air through her lips to form words. I was having a busy day at work and didn't have the patience for her tired voice. It slowed me down and annoyed me. I couldn't imagine anyone being so tired. It struck me as a little dramatic. I should have just kept my mouth shut. I knew better. Yet for some reason, I couldn't keep quiet.

Later that night, I asked her, "Were you being dramatic or were you really that tired?" She asked me to repeat the question. She couldn't believe her ears. The question was that shocking.

She responded that she never felt so tired in her life and that she didn't appreciate me calling her dramatic. I explained that I didn't *mean* to call her dramatic. I just wanted to understand if she was that tired. She told me that she couldn't believe I'd ask her such a stupid question. Her tone screamed, "You insensitive dumbass!" I felt bad that I hurt her feelings. And now I understood that she *was* that tired.

How a pregnant woman feels should never be questioned.

If you have the urge to question her emotions, reactions, or level of drama, share it with me or share it with a stranger—better yet, tell your dog. (If you don't have one, then get one, so you have a dog to tell.)

The third time around, I've become an expert at listening to her talk about her aches and pains. I just say, "I'm sorry you're so uncomfortable." The first trimester sucked all the energy out of her. The second trimester made her feel bigger and more uncomfortable. The third trimester was a hodgepodge of symptoms, aches, and pains. Running to the bathroom, getting kicked by the baby, and dealing with the issues described in Tip #34 and Tip #40 will give your partner reason to be completely, fall-on-her-face, never-so-tired-in-her-life exhausted.

If your partner is working while pregnant or taking care of other kids at home, she might have nothing left for you when she gets home. She'll need help with meals, cleaning, and the things she used to do (assuming she did these things). For guys who are used to sitting on their asses, this can be shocking. Just appreciate that every time you help her out, it will make her feel that much less tired and more supported. Bonus: she might even find time and energy for pregnancy sex.

THE BOTTOM LINE:

I'm tired, but I can't tell anyone either. Thanks for listening.

Tip #40
THE SNORING, RESTLESS PREGNANT WOMAN: Like Sleeping on the Tarmac of the Airport

THE TIP:

They should call the couch a bed because it's where you'll do some of your best sleeping.

THE STORY:

I've never been a good sleeper in a room with noise. My wife was a great silent sleeper, the secret to our marriage. She never snored until she got pregnant. Then she would constantly shift around. She would go to the bathroom several times a night. I didn't complain. I got up and slept on the couch because it was the only place I could sleep. We never talked about it. It was like my place was on the couch, and no one needed to talk about it. She didn't miss me. I enjoyed my couch.

—Gary, sons, six months and two

***

Sleeping in the same bed with a pregnant woman is like sleeping on an airplane in the middle seat in front of a kid who keeps kicking you. It's a series of constant interruptions. You might get some sleep, but it's broken sleep. And it's not like you

> I'm a stomach sleeper and need to be a side sleeper. So I bought a long pregnancy pillow so I don't roll over on my back. He uses it more than me.
>
> *—Stacey, twenty-five weeks pregnant*

AND NOW, ANOTHER ACCIDENTAL ASSHOLE MOMENT

Early one morning last week, hubby was snoring something fierce and I was trying to get back to sleep. I whacked him in the arm to make him stop, to which he responded, "I can't help it." I replied, "I know, but hitting you makes it stop." In his current state of sleep, he said, "Maybe you should go sleep on the couch." Dumbfounded, I told him that was the stupidest thing he's ever said, and he asked, "Why?" I said, "Really? You're telling your eight-months pregnant wife to go sleep on the couch because YOU are snoring?!" Later that night, I brought up the conversation, asking him if he remembered what he told me that morning. He kind of bust out laughing when I explained he had no memory since he was still "sleeping."

—Jessica, daughter, three, thirty-three weeks pregnant

can change where you sleep or complain about your pregnant partner's sleep habits. However bad it is for you, trust that sleeping is harder for her. And here's why:

- The expanding uterus puts pressure on the bladder. Constant pressure on the bladder can mean constant runs to the bathroom and constantly disrupted sleep (hopefully she will close the door).
- The growing baby will put pressure on the spine and

the circulatory system. Therefore women can't sleep on their stomachs or their backs late in the pregnancy. This can mean a lot of tossing and turning.

- Your sleeping partner will constantly be getting kicked and poked by the baby in the middle of the night. The moving baby can keep her up.
- Roughly a quarter of pregnant women will snore—these are the same women who didn't snore before they were pregnant (sleeping on her side and using breathing strips can help).
- Pregnant women get hungry at all times of the day and night. Sometimes she will wake up and need food. If she's too big or tired to get to the kitchen, you might need to get her some nourishment.
- Terrible leg cramps can keep her up at night—moaning and groaning (stretching, heat, and straightening the knee and flexing the foot can help).
- Pregnancy congestion may cause her to sneeze, snort, and blow her nose at all hours of the night.
- Heartburn, gas, constipation, aches, pains, general discomfort, anxiety, and hormones can make sleeping elusive for her and for you.

If she does wake you up, go back to sleep or quietly move to the couch (unless moving to the couch would upset or insult your partner; in that situation, ask if she'd like you to quietly move to the couch).

THE BOTTOM LINE:
Keep food and water next to her bed. It will save you a trip in the middle of the night.

Looking for more great features to help you prep for your new arrival? Get the *Dad's Expecting Too* week-by-week pregnancy tracker, designed for dads and their partners, along with weekly updates about baby, your partner, and you at DadsExpectingToo.com.

✳✳✳

To get the latest news, info, facts, and stats for new and expecting parents, follow @DadsExpecting on Twitter and check out the Dad's Expecting Facebook Page at www.Facebook.com /DadsExpecting.

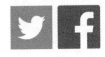

6

THE MIND OF THE PREGNANT WOMAN

And the Expectant Mother Thong
(Note: I'll explain the thong on page 195.)

It's hard enough for a man to understand the mind of a not-pregnant woman. Wait until she's pregnant. She may say, do, and feel things she's never done, said, or felt before. She might not even know why or when it's happening. This section will help you know what to say and do, but more importantly, what *never* to say or do.

THE TIP:

Some pregnancies can be smooth and easy. It's not at all as terrible or difficult as she thought it might be.

THE STORY:

My due date is tomorrow. I've had a really easy pregnancy the whole time. I feel lucky. I haven't had a lot to complain about. I think I've been even more relaxed while I'm pregnant as opposed to not pregnant. I've been learning to have perspective and appreciate how great life is. It's kind of a riot watching my body change. I love it. Every step of the way, I didn't know what was happening. I was expecting to be bigger, but I wasn't. I was expecting to get sick, but I didn't. I was expecting to be more uncomfortable, but I wasn't. My husband and I just look at each other and shake our heads in disbelief because all we ever heard was how hard and difficult pregnancy is. We're surprised by how much we've enjoyed it. Do we know anyone who has had a smooth and easy pregnancy and didn't complain about it? Not that I can think of. I feel like I'm an anomaly. It's been a breeze.

—*Amy, forty weeks pregnant*

***

I was surprised at how many people didn't like being pregnant. I loved it. I couldn't figure out what was so awful about it. I felt cheated because my baby was born a month early.

—*Mandy, son, two months*

Forget whipping out your empathy belly—some women absolutely love being pregnant. And for the women who don't love it, there's nothing wrong with reminding them of the perks. Pick and choose your favorites and share at the right time:

- Pregnant women must eat more and gain weight. Delicious.
- People hold doors open, give up their seats, and let them cross the street.
- Pregnant women get priority seating.
- Pregnant women get positive attention from men.
- Pregnant women get to do a lot of shopping. A lot of women love shopping.
- Pregnant women can get better parking spots. Many busy malls reserve parking for pregnant and new moms. (There are no spots for new dads—now isn't that the most sexist thing ever?)
- Pregnant women get thick hair, glowing skin, and strong nails (usually).
- Pregnant women can forget whatever they want and blame it on being pregnant.
- Pregnant women can pick the movies they want to see, eat where they want, and go home whenever they get tired.
- Pregnant women get large breasts without surgery. (This is something women with smaller breasts may enjoy.)
- Pregnant women get the entire bed to themselves (snoring, restlessness, gas, and constantly urinating tend to clear out a room).

- Pregnant women get gifts (jewelry, maternity clothes, massages, flowers, and other special treatments).
- Pregnant women have a place to rest their hands and somewhere to place snacks (M&Ms).
- Pregnant women create life—that's awesome.

THE BOTTOM LINE:

With so many perks to pregnancy, it's hard to imagine how a woman could complain…

Tip #42
THE HORMONAL PREGNANT WOMAN: Swinging on Her Moods Like a Monkey

THE TIP:

Hormonal pregnant woman (gunpowder) + clueless man (spark) = explosive situation.

THE STORY:

My wife told me she didn't like the taste of Morningstar Broccoli Cheddar Veggie Bites. I thought I was doing her a favor by trying to get them out of the house. I made them for my lunch, thinking I was doing good because now she wouldn't have to see them in the freezer. I was all proud of myself when she walked into the kitchen. I had a big smile on my face and told her, "Good news, I decided

> When I would get very angry or cry, he didn't understand. I had to keep reminding him it was only hormonal.
>
> —Susan, son, four, thirty-six weeks pregnant

to make the rest of the broccoli bites to get them out of the freezer!" She had a stunned look that turned into rage. She was *so* angry that I could be *so* inconsiderate to make these while she was in the house. The smell alone made her want to vomit. She already had a nauseating day, and this put her over the edge. She burst into tears and stormed away. I just stood there with my Morningstar Broccoli Cheddar Veggie Bites, wondering what the hell just happened.

—Brad, son, two, twenty-six weeks pregnant

***

Living with a pregnant partner can be like walking on eggshells. I know because I tried walking on eggshells as part of the research for this book, but when I put eggshells on the clean kitchen floor, my pregnant wife got pissed. So I figured out that even if you try to walk on eggshells, you'll upset a pregnant woman. That's how sensitive things can be.

The flood of estrogen, progesterone, and other hormones coursing through her veins can make even the simplest

GETTING COMFORTABLE IN YOUR EXPECTANT THONG

1. Accept that this time in life will be naturally uncomfortable and unpredictable.
2. Look in the mirror and acknowledge the things hanging out of your thong.
3. Turn to people, places, and resources to help you get comfortable with the uncomfortable, instead of overreacting and heightening situations. Then you'll be able to focus inward, look outward, and be more supportive, compassionate, and empathetic.

conversations troublesome. For example, the other day my wife was telling me how ridiculously tired she was feeling. I said, "Sweetie, why don't you take a nap?" She replied, "I don't want to take a nap. I have things to do." I answered, "Then don't take a nap." She snapped back, "Don't tell me what I can do! I know I don't need to take a nap." I was tempted to tell her, "Clearly, you're overtired and need a nap." But implying that she was crabby would only increase her level of crabbiness, and that's not going to make my life any better.

As a third-time expectant father, I know better. I know this wasn't really her—it was the hormones affecting her. Hormones are to blame for the road rage, crying during commercials, lack of patience, and general unpredictable nature. At least, this has been my experience (not all women react this way). I genuinely feel bad that hormones cause her to say, do, and feel things over which she has little control. Sometimes she doesn't even realize why she's doing something. It's only after the hormonal haze passes that she finds clarity. She always gets her feet back on the ground and makes things better.

The hormonal pregnant woman tends to:

- Cry more often
- Cry more easily
- Become angry faster
- Become impatient quickly
- Lose (or misplace) her sense of humor
- Need and want more attention
- Be more critical of people around her
- Be more critical of herself
- Hide her feelings
- Feel confused and out of control
- Lash out at strangers (this can be fun to watch)

Understand that the things you said and did before she got pregnant may affect her differently now. A joke that was once funny before pregnancy can become insulting and insensitive. A gentle touch can send her into a rage. A favorite move that you do in bed might get you kicked out of bed.

On top of the hormonal changes, another reason she might be extra sensitive is that, as a first-time mom, she's likely to be uncomfortable in the Expectant Mother Thong.

Let me explain the Expectant Mother Thong.

Throughout our lives, we take on different roles. Some of these roles are more uncomfortable than others. The more uncomfortable the role, the more we feel as if we're standing

THINGS THAT WILL SEND HER OVER THE EDGE

1. Dismissing her feelings ("You're just hormonal, you'll get over it.")
2. Referring to her as moody, crabby, bitchy, etc.
3. Not listening to her and not acknowledging her feelings

THINGS THAT WILL BRING HER BACK FROM THE EDGE

1. Being patient
2. Giving her room to feel however she feels
3. Regularly reminding her of her best qualities
4. Doing something out of the ordinary for her
5. Taking her out on a date (movie, dinner, coffee)
6. Listening and being there
7. Connecting her to professional help

on a crowded beach, totally exposed and completely vulnerable. When you're uncomfortable in your thong, little things can set you off. Innocent jokes are seen as insulting jabs. A helpful comment isn't so helpful. A friendly gesture can be seen as insensitive and mean.

Take a pregnant woman who is gaining weight, but doesn't like her new size—she's literally uncomfortable in her thong. When she's this uncomfortable, any comment, look, or touch she doesn't like can be misinterpreted. For example, that loving pat on her rear end can be interpreted as a signal that her butt is too big, when in reality you were just trying to be affectionate. The more uncomfortable she feels, the more likely she is to snap. Hormones just exacerbate these feelings.

But it's not just women. Expectant fathers aren't always comfortable in the Expectant Father Thong (sorry about the image). With all the changes we're facing, it's hard not to take our pregnant partner's words and actions personally. Knowing that being uncomfortable is normal and natural allows you to be much more understanding and patient. (**Note:** Everyone tends to be much more comfortable in their thongs the second time around—and that makes navigating through the pregnancy so much easier. But it takes walking through the unknown to get to this point.)

Should she freak out, cry, get angry, or have an irrational outburst, be forgiving and understand that it's not you. She's just trying to figure out what the hell is happening with her mind and body. It's just hard to not take some things personally when everyone is standing around in their thongs.

THE BOTTOM LINE:
When her moods swing, get out of the way.

Tip #43
THE STRONG PREGNANT WOMAN: We Are Not the Superior Sex

THE TIP:

When you think she's being strong, tell her. Women like this.

THE STORY:

Throughout my pregnancy, my husband would tell me how strong I was and how much he appreciated what I was going through for us. I had a natural birth with no medication. He was there the whole time, holding my hand through the contractions and the pushing. I didn't even realize it, but he later told me that I squeezed his hand so hard that it hurt him for days following the delivery. Seeing the pain on my face and feeling how tightly I squeezed his hand made him realize that he could never go through what I went through. He kept telling me this. Having him tell me this made me feel like he understood, and that was a great feeling.

—Elena, daughters, five and eight

***

We are *not* the superior sex.

Let me explain: we can't create, nurture, and push a kid out of our penis.

With advances in technology and medicine, women don't need men. If women wanted to take over the world, they could store our sperm and eliminate men (or keep us in cages). Considering we each have millions of sperm, women could inseminate themselves and create a world totally dominated by women. It's nice of women *not* to do this, but if we pissed them off enough, they could. The reality that women could be self-sufficient is probably one reason why men have tried to dominate and control women. It's threatening to know that we can be wiped out and the human race could still survive, even thrive, and smell good too (women smell better).

The awesome physical and emotional strength of your partner might hit you during the ultrasound. It might sink in when you feel a kick in her belly. It might become obvious when she vomits twenty times in twenty days (and still works, makes dinner, and makes love to you). It might strike during the final push or after the baby's first cry. Where, when, and how it hits you can't be predicted, but at some point you will realize it. Women are emotionally and physically strong—it's awesome (and scary in a way), and they like to hear about it. It makes them feel good.

They like to hear that we can't do it. They like to know that we get it. It makes them feel appreciated and acknowledged. There's a good reason why men don't do the birthing in the family. Men can't even manage their emotions after a few drinks. Imagine a dude, totally sober, carrying twins at thirty-two weeks. He'd be beating up everyone so they could understand and feel his pain. That's why men don't get pregnant.

THE BOTTOM LINE:
Women could freeze our sperm, wipe us out, and inseminate themselves for millions of years to come. Be nice.

Tip #44
THE CRANKY PREGNANT WOMAN: This Time, We Are Partly to Blame

THE TIP:

The most helpful thing you can do is not snap back, even when she's at her worst. Instead, tell her that you love her.

THE STORY:

After having two kids and having gone through this before, he knows where the crankiness is coming from and doesn't let it upset him. He knows that I get impatient, tired, sensitive, and exhausted. When I snap at him, he just lets it go most of the time. Once in a while, he will tell me when I'm being a bitch, but generally, he doesn't fight with me. The other day, I sent him a snippy email, and he responded back to me, "I love you." Another time this week, I was helping him with some contract work (I'm an attorney, now full-time mom), and I called him up and started yelling at him that his secretary needs to proof his work because it wasn't professional. He just let it go. Even when I'm at my worst, he doesn't argue or fight.

—Bridgette, daughters, three and one and a half, sixteen weeks pregnant

***

The cranky pregnant woman is much different from the cranky NOT-pregnant woman. The big difference? *You* got her pregnant. This means that being cranky is not just her problem—it's yours too. Once the crankiness is attached to being pregnant, you take partial ownership.

Some women will want you to feel their crankiness. This might manifest itself in wanting to make you cranky, taking the crankiness out on you, or just making you do something that will take her mind off her own crankiness.

Thankfully, there is a five-step plan to confronting her crankiness:

1. Focus your attention on her: do not multitask; no texting, no phone; give her your full attention.
2. Listen quietly, intently, and patiently: make eye contact, but *never* roll your eyes.
3. Sympathize with her crankiness: apply the nonforgiveness apology (see Tip #46).
4. Ask what you can do to help: be genuine when asking and be willing to actually do something if she has a suggestion.
5. Stay out of her way: give her space to be cranky (it will pass).

Let's look at how these steps would work in a real-life scenario.

When my wife enters the room and gives off that cranky vibe, I stop what I'm doing and focus my attention on her. When she speaks, I'll listen quietly, intently, and patiently. If she explains that she's exhausted, I'll respond with, "I'm so sorry you're tired. That sucks." By acknowledging her crankiness, she knows that I'm aware of the problem. I also acknowledge that it sucks that she has to go through it and I don't have to go through it. Next, I will ask what I can do for her. This accomplishes two things: (1) It means that I'm willing to make an effort to help, and (2) If she says "There's nothing you can do," it allows me the opportunity to watch TV, play video games, work out, or go online without turning into an accidental asshole. All that said, sometimes none of these things will help, but attempting to help is all we can be expected to do.

Should you find yourself in an argument with a cranky pregnant woman, winning isn't the goal. It's about ending the argument as quickly as possible. (Refer to Tip #46: The Irrational Pregnant Woman for how to diffuse the situation and give yourself permission to be wrong and still be right.) And whatever you do, never joke about her mood (at least not to her). Even if she finds it funny one day, she might not find it funny the next (see Tip #42: The Hormonal Pregnant Woman). This includes *not* joking even if she jokes first. Her joke might be a trap; do not get caught in it.

If her crankiness and irritability don't stop, consider pointing your partner in the direction of a therapist or discussing her mood with her care provider. The crankiness and irritability can be symptomatic of a deeper issue like prepartum or postpartum depression (see Tip #49).

THE BOTTOM LINE:

You got her pregnant, so you're partly responsible for her crankiness (I know that's ridiculous, but it's true).

Tip #45
THE ANGRY PREGNANT WOMAN: It's Not about Us, It's about Them

THE TIP:

Some pregnant women are just angry and there's little we can do about it.

THE STORY:

During my first trimester, I was having a hard time with smells. He'd come home from work and cook dinner on our George Foreman grill—usually grilled chicken with vegetables and some type of noodles. Some nights, he'd do it all himself. The smell of chicken on the grill nauseated me. Afterward, he didn't clean the grill right away so the smell would linger. I wouldn't tell him because I wanted to be angry. The testosterone levels got to me; it was easy to go from zero to sixty. It wasn't anyone's fault I was pissy, but I often just wanted to simmer in my anger. I wanted to feel bad for myself. I was going through all these changes during the first trimester and I wanted to feel like I was the only one who was ever pregnant—like me and my pregnancy were the only things going on in this world. I was focused on me. So when the grill sat there, dirty and smelly, I wouldn't say a word. And then when he'd come home the next day, I'd clean it and tell him how angry I was about it.

—Effie, thirty-nine weeks pregnant

***

If cranky is a simmer, angry is a boil.

If you've done nothing wrong, recognize that her lashing out at you could just be a product of her being uncomfortable, unhappy, and out of control. It could be her body, her mind, her identity, or other issues bubbling to the surface. When people are uncomfortable in their thongs, they will often get angry.

Given that she has so little control over her life during pregnancy, getting angry and watching you get angry might be one of the last things she can control. While allowing her to get you angry might mean giving her what she wants, there's only so much an expectant father should be expected to do in order to make her happy—being a verbal punching bag isn't one of them.

And I want to be clear—you have every right to be respected. If you're not being respected, make sure you tell her (pick a quiet moment to share your feelings).

Now, if you've done something wrong (like leaving a dirty smelly grill sitting on the counter) and she has good reason to be angry, don't defend what you've done. Don't make excuses. That will just make her angrier. Admit your mistake. Wait until she cools down. If you insist on continuing to make her angry, this might be *you* exerting control over the situation because your life is so out of control. And that's just not a nice thing to do to your pregnant partner.

Assuming you're innocent, talk to her after she cools down. Ask what you can do to make her happy. If she's always angry, point her in the direction of professional care. Anger and irritability can be normal, but they can also be a symptom of deeper issues.

THE BOTTOM LINE:

While she might get upset, verbal and emotional abuse are NEVER acceptable—pregnant or not. If you find she's stepping over the line, wait until she's cool and calm and explain what is making you uncomfortable. If it doesn't stop, get away and then find a couple's therapist to help.

Tip #46
THE IRRATIONAL PREGNANT WOMAN: Letting Her Be Right Even If She's Wrong

THE TIP:

If you get yelled at for something irrational, give her time to realize she's wrong—she should come around.

THE STORY:

My wife was having a bad day and I wanted to help her out. I have honestly never done dishes before. I washed the plates and loaded everything in the dishwasher while she took a nap. When she woke up, she saw the way I had loaded the dishwasher and said, "I can't believe how obnoxiously you loaded the dishwasher." She thought I should have loaded it with more dishes before running the cycle. I thought she was lucky that I took the time to load the dishwasher. After bitching me out, she went back to whatever it was that she was doing. It took her about eight hours to realize

> You just can't win. So just don't try. Just be wrong and be happy about it.
>
> —*Mark, sons, ten months and two and a half*

that she was wrong. I didn't argue with her at the time. What's the point? When doing nice things for your wife, make sure you do them the right way. To this day, we joke about the "obnoxious loading" of the dishwasher. I have yet to put dishes in the dishwasher since.

—Jim, daughter, two months, son, three

***

Arguing with a pregnant woman in the midst of an irrational outburst is like arguing with a drunk on dime beer night. You will never win.

I started writing this book with fading memories of our first and second pregnancies. I'm now in the midst of the third trimester of our third pregnancy. It's all fresh—almost too fresh. While my wife is dealing with a lot of the same issues, the third time around is different for me. I'm now completely comfortable with the concept: *I don't have to be right to be right.* What I mean is that I don't need her to tell me that I'm correct to know I'm right. I'm not saying that I'm always right. In fact, I'm an expert at being wrong. But when she is wrong, I don't need her to see it my way; *I can be right and wrong.*

Sometimes I'll apologize for upsetting her even if she's wrong. I use the "nonforgiveness apology" to diffuse the situation. This form of apology acknowledges that she's upset and that you understand that she's upset. You say, "I'm sorry if I upset you," and that's it. It's the same as her having an ache or pain and you saying, "I'm sorry you're so uncomfortable." You're not seeking forgiveness—just offering compassion.

Truly, when I'm right and she's wrong, I do feel bad for her. About 99 percent of the time, she apologizes later, once her head clears. If something really bothers me and she doesn't apologize, I'll revisit the issue at a different time and in a different location. Then I'll explain myself and leave it at that. Other times, I'll just let it go because I know she's pregnant and dealing with a lot.

Now, I'm not saying you should always let things go (that's called being abused). It's important to talk about the big issues, but it's just as important to pick the right time and the right place to discuss them. As a first-time expectant father, you might think you have a right to be right. But all that does is make you wrong. As a rule: upsetting a tired, exhausted, and overwhelmed pregnant woman is wrong—even if you know you're right.

THE BOTTOM LINE:

Sometimes being right means giving her permission to think you're wrong even when it's glaringly obvious that you're right.

Tip #47
THE SCARED PREGNANT WOMAN: You'd Be Scared Too if It Were in You

THE TIP:

Remind her of all the things she's doing right. Keep reassuring her that everything will be okay. She might need to hear it over and over again.

THE STORY:

The fear of the unknown was the worst. For a while, a part of me believed a C-section might be easier because I understand surgery and can relate to it. Having a C-section would mean not doing the pushing and going through labor. In retrospect, I know how much better it is to deliver vaginally. My recovery has been far easier than friends and family members who have had C-sections. One thing that helped me: When I told him that I was kind of scared, he would tell me that I was doing everything I could to prepare, and he would actually run down the list of all the things I had done right. He'd remind me that it was going to be okay. Hearing that I had done everything I could do to have a healthy pregnancy reassured me. The anxiety I felt before giving birth was far worse than the actual birth.

—*Kate, son, two weeks*

***

My wife and I would be walking, eating, or running errands and she would just bust out:

"How can a baby come out of my vagina?"

"My pants are tight. I hate it! I hate it! I hate it!"

"I'm too young to be a mom. Aren't I too young?"

Until she's gone through pregnancy and childbirth, it's

I left the prenatal class crying because I realized that although it was quite easy and fun for the baby to get in there, it wasn't going to be so much fun to get it out. My husband was very comforting and kept telling me that once I actually went into labor, the only thing I'd care about was getting that baby out, and he was right.

—*Jenn, daughter, two*

She's not the first, and she won't be the last. That's what I told my wife when she got scared.
—Franco, father of one

impossible to know what it will be like, for her and for you. A lot of it is scary. That's what it means to fear the unknown.

She might be scared of the pain, labor and delivery, complications, miscarriage, finances, the doctor, caring for the baby, getting a C-section, pushing, being able to nurse, pooping while pushing (a common fear), the possibility that her body will turn you off (especially after pooping while pushing), what happens after the baby is born, your marriage, parenting issues, and everything else that will happen as you continue this journey into the unknown.

Here are some things you can do to calm her:

1. Acknowledge that she's scared. Before telling her it's going to be okay, tell her that you understand. Letting her feel scared will help her get beyond it. Shutting it down will just aggravate her.
2. Remind her that being scared is normal. All these changes, the prospect of pain, the medical issues that come with being pregnant, and the responsibility are all very scary. If she wasn't scared, something would be wrong.
3. Remind her that this is something billions of women have done before. If it were so terrible, they wouldn't keep having children. Having a child connects her to all the women who have done it before her. Encourage her to reach out to other moms who have been there and done it. She's not the first and won't be the last.
4. Encourage her to talk to her caregiver about her questions and fears. Suggest that she make a list (or you can

make one) of the things that concern her. If she can't talk to her doctor, she needs a new doctor or a therapist.

5. Participate in the pregnancy with her—prenatal appointments, birthing classes, shopping, reading her books. Your participation will help her feel like she's not alone and that you're in it together.

6. Consider getting a doula (a doula is a birth coach who will help reassure her before, during, and after the birth). (See Tip #4.)

7. Remind her that she's beautiful again and again. She needs to hear it…again and again.

8. Listen to her and be there for her. Just being there quietly will make her feel secure and safe. Silence can speak volumes.

9. Do something fun together. Keep her busy doing things she loves so she can focus on something other than the fear.

For me, the hardest parts of seeing her so scared was that it scared me. I didn't want to be scared. But once I allowed myself to feel it (see Tip #3), it made it easier to listen and allow her to feel these same feelings.

Once you can get comfortable with the uncomfortable and allow yourself to *not* always know what's going to happen, you can focus your energy on the things you can control. Being there for each other is one of the most powerful things you *can* control.

THE BOTTOM LINE:

If she's scared, help her see that billions of women have done this for millions of years and they keep doing it.

Tip #48
THE NESTING PREGNANT WOMAN: Cleaning House with Your Toothbrush

THE TIP:

If she talks about hanging a large chandelier in the nursery, it's time to intervene.

THE STORY:

I was obsessed with the nursery. I would come home from work and do nothing but search websites, cut and paste pictures into a PowerPoint slide show, and design the baby's room. I picked out an over-the-top chandelier (we live in a condo with low ceilings), a beautiful antique-looking iron crib (that cost $40,000), and gorgeous bedding ($1,500+). My husband would come downstairs and watch me. He wasn't pushy; he let me do it for a while. I would sit in my pajamas, eat ice cream, and decorate this fantasy room for hours. The crazy part was that I knew I was having a boy but insisted on creating a girl's room. This went on for about five weeks. Then one day, my husband left to work out and run errands. When he came back five hours later, I was still online right where he left me. He looked me straight in the eyes and told me this had to stop. Now I laugh thinking about that moment. That's when it sunk in that I was obsessed with a girl's room and I wasn't even having a girl. I realized it was stupid and stopped.

—*Christine, son, three*

***

Your partner won't actually build a nest. (If she does build a nest with twigs and leaves in your home, point her in the direction of professional help.) Nesting refers to the primal urge to prepare the home for the arrival of the new baby. The feeling usually hits in the second trimester and continues until the baby comes home to the nest.

Nesting is about control—not cleaning and organizing. Control is a constant theme throughout pregnancy. Having so little control means exerting control over things she can impact (your home, you, etc.). The Internet has opened up a whole new outlet that allows women to spend hundreds of hours searching for the perfect nursery items (it's futuristic nesting).

Nesting for a man means doing the things you've put off for years—things you agreed to do, but never actually believed you would have to do. When the nesting hits, she will become a cleaning-and-organizing machine, and she'll enlist you. Not participating can be interpreted as not wanting to be involved in the life of your new child (a big leap, I know). And the nesting instinct can strike her at the worst times—in the midst of the playoffs, on a Saturday night, after work, in the middle of lovemaking, or right before dinner.

If you're around when the urge hits her but don't want to participate, it doesn't matter. When you see your pregnant partner in her ninth month carrying a bookshelf up the stairs, you'll find the energy to help.

When it happens, she will start throwing away things (sometimes things that don't need to be thrown away or things you still want). She might start disinfecting and scrubbing with a toothbrush (yes, my wife). She will arrange and rearrange. She might paint or do a project while you're at work. (Tell her to avoid paints and other noxious fumes—the chemicals in some paints can be harmful for pregnant women to inhale.)

The best advice is to talk about this before it hits her. (Try starting the conversation in the first trimester.) Put together a plan so that when her nesting instinct kicks in, you can remind her of the plan. Include a timeline as part of the plan, and stick to the plan or do things ahead of schedule. Then, when the urge hits, instead of getting pulled into her nesting, you can remind her that you plan to do it according to the timeline. But then again, she might say, "Screw your timeline" (that's some mouth on her) and grab the bookshelf. There might be no stopping her.

THE BOTTOM LINE:

She can't be trusted alone with paint, power tools, and heavy furniture. Stay close while she's nesting.

THE TIP:

If a guy sees his partner not playing with the kids or interacting, not getting out of bed, and not being herself, *he needs to get her help.*

THE STORY:

My doctor gave my husband and my mom her card. She told them to call if they thought I needed help. Carrying twins meant I was at greater risk. When the twins were first born, I was happy and excited in the hospital. They were healthy preemies. We left the hospital without both of them and that was very difficult. Once my first baby came home, I was tired, but I wasn't sad or depressed. Once the second came home, that's when the depression hit me. They were so needy, and I had no time for myself. I'd wake up, feed them, feed myself, and pump (I never produced enough milk for a full bottle). Somewhere in between, I'd brush my teeth and get dressed. After I fed them, I wasn't that interested in playing with them or tickling them. It was like being in school and having to go to class. Every time they would wake up, I would go to feed them—I didn't want to, but I had to. They took forever to eat because they were premature, and feeding is so slow. They also had terrible reflux and cried for hours on end.

I didn't talk to my friends about these feelings because I didn't want them to know. I wasn't ashamed; I just didn't want them to think that I had mental problems. None of my friends told me they went through postpartum depression, and they couldn't relate to having twins. My husband was so helpful, but he was very worried about their health as preemies. Inside I was thinking, "I feel like crap and he's worried about their health."

When I went to the doctor for my six-week checkup, I told her what was happening and that I went to Target to do some shopping and didn't want to come home. She said,

PERINATAL DEPRESSION

Perinatal depression (depression during pregnancy) is so hard to diagnose because so many of the symptoms associated with it are a normal part of pregnancy. Again, this is where having a relationship with your partner's caregiver and attending appointments can be so helpful.

"You're the eleventh case of someone not wanting to come home from Target." The doctor prescribed some medication, and about three weeks later, things began to get better. I started to want to interact more and be there for my girls. It's still hard for me at times, but I'm grateful I was able to get help and never endangered myself or my girls.

—*Anne, twin daughters, twenty months*

✳✳✳

She might get depressed. Watch for it.

About 10 to 15 percent of you will have a partner who will suffer from perinatal (during pregnancy) and/or postpartum (postpregnancy) depression any time from a month

BABY BLUES OR DEPRESSION?

The baby blues can happen in the days right after childbirth and normally go away within a few days to a week. A new mother can experience sudden mood swings, sadness, crying spells, loss of appetite, and sleeping problems, and feel irritable, restless, anxious, and lonely. Symptoms are not severe and treatment isn't needed. Symptoms that linger more than a few days need to be discussed with your physician.

to a year after childbirth (source: National Institutes of Health). And more than one in ten of YOU reading this will suffer from post-partum depression (PPD).

Your partner might be in pain and never tell you. She might have thoughts of hurting herself or the baby and keep them a secret. The best news is that treatment is available (medical and nonmedical), but she needs to get help to get better. And that means you need to be involved and aware.

If you aren't the primary caregiver and work long hours, travel a lot, or aren't around for hours at a time following the birth (up to a year) and you sense a problem, have your mom, mother-in-law, family, or her friends stop in and visit to make sure she's okay. If she exhibits any of the symptoms listed in this section or you feel that something isn't right, talk to her caregiver and get the name of a mental health professional.

A lot of women suffering from PPD will *not* seek help. She will call the doctor when she gets a cramp, but when the symptoms of depression surface, she'll keep it a secret. If at any point your partner exhibits any of the following symptoms (during or after pregnancy) and the symptoms last longer than two weeks, make sure you let her caregiver know. Here are some signs to watch for:

- Feeling restless or irritable
- Feeling sad, hopeless, and overwhelmed
- Crying a lot
- Having no energy or motivation
- Eating too little or too much
- Sleeping too little or too much
- Trouble focusing, remembering, or making decisions
- Feeling worthless and guilty
- Loss of interest or pleasure in activities she used to enjoy
- Withdrawal from friends and family
- Having headaches, chest pains, heart palpitations (fast heartbeats or skipping heartbeats), or hyperventilation (fast and shallow breathing)
- Not interacting with or showing interest in the baby
- Fear of being alone with the baby
- Expressing thoughts of hurting herself or the baby

WHAT EVERY EXPECTANT FATHER MUST KNOW:

> Try to get a psychologist involved as soon as possible. When she doesn't want to get involved with her children, that's a sign she needs help.
>
> —*Steve, father of two girls*

1. Bring up the risk of perinatal and postpartum depression early in the pregnancy. By helping your partner see that this is an illness that is *not* a reflection on how much she loves you or the baby,

POSTPARTUM PSYCHOSIS

In extremely rare cases—less than 1 percent of new mothers—women may develop something called postpartum psychosis. It usually occurs within the first few weeks after delivery. Symptoms may include refusing to eat, frantic energy, sleep disturbance, paranoia, and irrational thoughts. Women with postpartum psychosis usually need to be hospitalized.

(Source: The National Institutes of Health)

you help alleviate the shame. Treatment is available (medical and nonmedical). Men need to be good listeners, because if you don't hear her cries for help, you might miss her calling out for attention.

2. Sporadically check in with her during pregnancy and ask how she's feeling (you'll notice the doctor will do this if you go to appointments with her). It's way too easy to dismiss her moods and actions as hormonal. In reality, there could be more happening. If she's having a hard time, suggest she find a therapist she can talk to. Then once the baby is born, she will have built a relationship with someone she trusts. If you have to leave her at home alone, make sure people will be checking in and dropping by to visit.

3. Once the baby is born, encourage your partner to:

   1. Try to get rest—nap when the baby naps.
   2. Stop putting pressure on herself to do everything.

She should only do as much as she can and leave the rest!

3. Ask for your help with household chores and nighttime feedings. Ask you to bring the baby to her for feeding. Have a friend, family member, or professional support person help you in the home for part of the day.
4. Talk to your family and friends about how she is feeling.
5. Avoid spending a lot of time alone. Spend it with other moms, friends, and family.
6. Spend time alone with you.
7. Talk with other mothers, so she can learn from their experiences.
8. Join a support group for women with depression if she thinks she may have PPD.

IF YOUR PARTNER SUFFERS FROM PPD

Being a partner of a depressed spouse or significant other can be overwhelming. You have to take care of her, the baby, and yourself. As important as it is for her to get help, it's equally important for you to find a support network. Find a group or one-on-one therapy. Essentially, you become a single father caring for the baby and your partner. There are several groups and websites for men with partners who have PPD. Care may also be covered under insurance.

THE BOTTOM LINE:

With the right help and support, postpartum depression can have a happy ending.

7

SPOILING YOUR PREGNANT PARTNER

Helping Her Feel as Good as She Feels Big

Tip #50
DATING A PREGNANT WOMAN: This Would Be Your Partner

THE TIP:
Your date doesn't have to be expensive or fancy. Making the effort will let her know you think she's still hot.

THE STORY:
I was *not* excited about leaving the house late in my pregnancy for a big Saturday night on the town. Besides getting tired at 8:00 p.m., I felt big and disgusting. My clothes felt like a tent. I also didn't like spending money. One night in

particular, he surprised me and told me to get dressed up. I fought it the whole way. We got in the car and arrived at an inexpensive neighborhood Italian restaurant. He kept telling me how hot and beautiful I looked. I have no idea to this day if he was just saying it, but I didn't stop him. After dinner, we saw a movie—the last one we saw for another nine months. What made it so special was that he made the effort. It was like he was still attracted to me and wanted to be with me. Yes, he did have a couple of drinks but only because I gave him clearance. Let me tell you, he earned those drinks—I wasn't the easiest preggo.

—Ally, daughter, eleven months

***

Most likely, you've never dated a pregnant woman. Now's your chance.

Asking your significant other on a date shouldn't be intimidating. Given that she's pregnant, you know that she's not a virgin (so you might get lucky). One more bonus—she looks kind of different from when you met her. So in a way, it's like dating a whole new woman. It makes for an exciting night on the town.

Once the kid drops into your world, things will be dramatically different (yes, everyone tells you this). But life will actually change for the better (I know I keep

> When taking her out for a date, don't you dare even glance at that pretty thing on the other side of the room—especially after the baby is born when your wife really feels fat.
>
> *—Cathy, sons, four months and three and a half*

> When going out with a pregnant woman, respect her energy level and mood. If she doesn't want to be there, get out of Dodge. Make sure people aren't smoking nearby. She will be extremely sensitive to anything that might harm the baby.
> —Mike, son, three months

telling you this). That said, spending time together and doing things as a couple will take more effort and planning once you have a child. In a few months, going out will mean finding a babysitter, paying for that babysitter, and pumping milk so that the babysitter can feed the baby if your partner is breastfeeding. (You don't actually have to pump them unless she asks.) Seeing a movie will cost you the price of the tickets, an additional $10 to $15 an hour depending on where you live (that's what people in Chicago pay for a sitter), plus popcorn, candy, and something to drink.

Enjoy going out while it's easy, spontaneous, and cheap. Besides taking advantage of this window of opportunity to have fun together, making the effort demonstrates that you still love her and want to be around her. Some women get paranoid that you will take off to the store for milk and bread and never come home. Spending quality time together goes a long way toward focusing on your life as a couple. And just like when you were single, if you want to have sex, wining (not whining) and dining her can increase your chances (as long as you get home before 9:00 p.m.). Oh, and no wine for her.

Take her to dinner. Take her to a movie. Take her to a museum. Take her to a sporting event (park close and avoid making her walk to the upper deck). Take her to a concert (after week twenty-six, the baby can hear the music

RULES FOR TAKING HER OUT

1. Make sure she can physically fit wherever you are going.
2. Make sure you don't accidentally walk too fast and leave her behind.
3. Make sure there are bathrooms, food, and drink nearby.
4. Make sure you can leave at any time if she gets really tired or emotional.

—Maggie, daughter, twenty months, son, three months

too). Take her shopping for clothes. Take her to a spa for the day or night. Take her on a hike. Take her on a bike. Take her to an open mic (sorry for the rhyming sequence). Take her to another room in the house for a candlelight dinner you prepared (I mean, ordered in).

Take charge and make an effort to give her attention. The goal isn't to get some action (although it improves your chances). The goal is to have some fun; to remind her that she's beautiful; to shower her with attention; to remind her that she's loved; to help her laugh, relax, and have a good time together.

THE BOTTOM LINE:

Dating isn't about getting lucky—it's about showing her that you still think she's hot and attractive.

Tip #51
THE BABYMOON: A Getaway While You Can Get Away

THE TIP:

Go to a place where there are things to see—not people you need to see. Keep the travel time under two hours. Check with the doctor if your wife plans to have a glass of wine with dinner.

THE STORY:

We researched places to go and picked Washington, D.C. Some of the warmer spots were too far to fly to, and at thirty-two weeks pregnant, she didn't want to sit for too long. We flew into D.C. around midday. We ate at a place called Old Capitol Grill, right next to the Capitol—I highly recommend it. Her doctor said an occasional glass of wine was fine, so she looked at the menu and ordered the most expensive glass. She said, "If I'm going to have one glass, I'll have a good one." She didn't finish it—I did. We toured the Capitol, the Smithsonian, and a spy museum.

The trip was a last chance to spend an isolated weekend— just the two of us. We didn't know anyone there, and that was a nice thing. If we had traveled to a place where we knew friends or family, we might have felt an obligation to meet up with them. It was great because we don't know when the next vacation will be together—and it won't be

> We planned a trip to Laguna Beach, California, in the second trimester. We went swimming, ate, walked around town— nothing too strenuous. It was perfect.
>
> —Mandy, daughter, two months

THE CLIFFS RESORT'S "AND BABY MAKES THREE" PACKAGE FOR PARENTS-TO-BE

Before baby makes three, couples can enjoy their last romantic getaway as a twosome at The Cliffs Resort. This Pismo Beach vacation package allows you to relax and pamper yourselves with a massage for Mom and Dad. Enjoy a $50 dinner voucher at the award-winning restaurant Marisol. Take in your last uninterrupted movie with the Muffin Goddess's Baby Cakes. This romantic Pismo Beach vacation package includes:

- Overnight luxury accommodations
- Tote bag with baby blanket
- Sparkling cider
- Muffin Goddess's Baby Cakes
- Two fifty-minute massage treatments
- $50 dinner voucher
- Movie
- Breakfast for Two

(Source: www.cliffsresort.com)

just the two of us! Right now, we're loving the experience of having our son in our lives and seeing all the changes.

—*Chris, son, two weeks*

***

Get away. Right now! Take this book and your pregnant partner and run.

Right now, it's soooo easy. Soon it won't be like this. It will either mean taking your baby with you or leaving him at home. If she's nursing, leaving the baby at home means pumping milk for a few days beforehand. If you take the baby with you, this means bringing an infant seat, a stroller, a crib or Pack 'n Play, formula, bottles, sleepers, a monitor, diapers, diaper cream, bath soap, a baby bathtub, toys, burp cloths, blankets, and a bunch of other stuff I'm sure I missed. It also means working a vacation around nap times, bedtime, and 3:00 a.m. feedings. The baby is the center of attention.

The point of the prebirth vacation is that you as a couple are the center of attention. So, even if you're on a tight budget, it would be nice to find a way to get away and spend some quality time together as a couple (not a threesome). Pick a night or two or three to get away. If you're on a budget, keep it local and drive to a bed-and-breakfast a couple hours from home. If you have a bigger budget, avoid planning a surprise safari to Kenya. That's too long to sit on an airplane, and she should be able to drink the water at your destination. Make it short and sweet. You might even opt for a package designed for pregnant couples (see the sidebar on the next page). If you do it right, the package will include a massage for two—which means you'll have to get one too. (**Note:** Also check with your caregiver to see if wine is on the menu. Ours said a few sips isn't a problem later in the pregnancy, but that's a personal judgment call.)

If planning a prebaby vacation, the best time is early into the second trimester (the honeymoon period of the pregnancy). Make sure it's a refundable trip or buy travel

THE W HOTEL'S "BABY ME" PACKAGE

Why not treat yourself to a luxurious getaway before the baby arrives? Go on a babymoon and celebrate your pregnancy with W Hotel's Baby Me package. Your experience includes:

- One pair of Baby Moccasins from W Hotels the Store for your baby to stroll around in style
- One Whoops Baby Onesie for snuggly moments
- Three items from the Womb Service Menu to satisfy your cravings
- One *Bump It Up: Transform Your Pregnancy into the Ultimate Style Statement* Book
- and a wonderful room you'll love!

(Source: www.starwoodpromos.com/whotelsbabyme/)

insurance just in case (check if pregnancy is insurable). Other things to keep in mind:

- Keep the travel time less than a few hours. Sitting can be uncomfortable and may turn her mood south (even when driving east, west, or north).
- If traveling by air late into the pregnancy (within a couple weeks of the due date), a doctor's letter might be required to board the plane.
- Always check with your care provider before making any travel plans.

- If driving, make sure the seat belt never goes over her belly—always low across her pelvic bone. Plan for a lot of stopping and anticipate pregnancy gas (see Tip #36).
- If going on a cruise, check the rules and regulations. Some cruise lines don't allow pregnant women beyond their 26th week on board. Bring a letter from the doctor just in case. Avoid first-trimester sailing—motion sickness plus morning sickness makes for a messy cabin.
- If traveling out of the country, check your health insurance plan to see if you're covered. If not, buy more insurance or change your destination.
- No drinking water at exotic ports of call outside the United States.
- If sitting for several hours, encourage her to walk around. Leg cramps, leg pain, and blood clots are possible complications.
- Consider getting travel insurance just in case she doesn't feel well enough to go (pregnant women can be unpredictable).

THE BOTTOM LINE:
You still haven't gone yet? Go!

Tip #52
THE PRENATAL RUBDOWN: Massaging Whatever She'll Let You Touch

THE TIP:
When giving her a pedicure, remember the base coat.

PREGNANCY Q & A

QUESTION: What can a man do to increase his chances of having sex?

ANSWER: Massage the mom's feet/shoulders. Run a bubble bath for her (not too hot). Tell her she looks amazing and sexy (but only if you're being honest—she'll know if you're insincere).

—Susan, pregnant, mother of one

QUESTION: The perfect gift for a pregnant woman?

ANSWER: A gift certificate for a pregnancy massage.

—Brittany, pregnant with number one

THE STORY:

I was on bed rest for several weeks, and my husband wanted to give me a pedicure. So he bought loofah scrubs, lotions, and a foot tub; I already had all the polishes and picked out bright red—a really hard color to use. I think he put on a football game while he did it; I like it so I didn't mind. He did what he thought a full pedicure would be. He started by putting my feet in a tub. Then he scrubbed my feet and massaged them for five minutes. He didn't do any of the clipping. I preferred that he not do that. Then he polished my toenails. He didn't apply a base coat, and I got one coat of red. I didn't say anything to him—I said "Thank you!" I've probably had worse, but I wouldn't be a repeat customer.

—*Renee, daughter, two months*

***

Women like to be touched. Men like to touch women. (That's what got you into this situation.)

If you've never given a massage, surprise her. It can be a two-minute massage or a twenty-minute one. Anything you can do is enough. The results will be dramatic. Massages are proven to improve circulation and the elasticity of the skin, decrease swelling, muscle fatigue, and stress, and help with sleeping. And touching can lead to other things. Besides connecting with her and possibly leading to action (see Chapter 8), it's a loving thing to do for her.

Encourage relatives or friends to buy her a massage gift certificate. You can also get her one for Valentine's Day, Mother's Day, or some special day that you make up to celebrate her.

If you have never given a massage and don't want to give one, then get her a gift certificate for a massage at a spa, health club, or hotel. Make sure they have a certified prenatal massage therapist on staff; certain pressure points of the body have been thought to trigger contractions. (Now, if you're in week forty-two and want to get this kid out, have the massage therapist touch all the right pressure points. Hell, have the therapist show you.)

If you want to give a massage and don't know how to give one or are afraid of hurting her, schedule a massage lesson. You can do it as a couple. My wife and I took a

> The best way to seduce a pregnant woman is to massage her sexy cankles, or in my case one cankle.
>
> —Jessica, daughter, three, thirty-three weeks pregnant

couples massage class before she got pregnant (and it enabled me to get her pregnant). We learned techniques such as effleurage (long strokes from the neck to lower back using the whole hand), petrissage (a rolling and squeezing action using the thumbs and fingers), and friction (moving the thumbs and fingers in little circles to penetrate the muscle).

If you wing it, proceed with light pressure and avoid the ankles until your due date; certain pressure points can cause premature labor. Make sure she's sitting or lying on her side (not on her stomach or back). If you want to get serious about this and make it an activity, turn down the lights, turn on mood music, bring out the massage oils, some candles, pillows, and towels, and go to town. The risk is that she enjoys it too much. Then she'll be expecting it all the time.

THE BOTTOM LINE:
Women love pregnancy massages.

Tip #53
MATERNITY CLOTHES: The Better She Feels, the Better Life Will Be

THE TIP:
Encourage her to buy maternity clothes. Buying bigger nonmaternity clothes to save money is a bad idea that will cost you in many other ways.

THE STORY:
When I was pregnant the first time, my husband thought it

would be a good idea to buy larger-size clothes instead of maternity clothes, which are only worn for nine months. The problem with bigger clothes is that they're not form-fitting; they just made me look like a gigantic cow. He would go to the discount rack and pick out something in a size 14 for

MONEY-SAVING TIP

Borrow clothes from friends and family. Search and buy on eBay and Craigslist. Shop at consignment stores. Get high-quality, lightly used clothes at a fraction of the cost.

me—I'm a size 6. We both thought it was silly to spend money on maternity clothes, but it's not a good feeling to feel ugly for nine months. During my second pregnancy, I splurged on maternity clothes. (When I say splurged, I mean shopping the sale at Gap Maternity.) I was so much happier. I felt pretty. I wanted to be more social because I looked nice. I was happier to go out and be with my friends. I felt less self-conscious. I looked cute. Because I was so much happier, it made being with me much easier. I wasn't nearly as crabby as I was with the first. The value of looking good and feeling good far exceeds the price, even if you will only wear it for nine months.

—Irene, daughters, seven and five, son, six months

I *forced* her to let me spend a few hundred bucks on her. For some reason, she was the one resisting.

—Todd, son, four months

✳✳✳

It's the best money she can spend. The better she looks, the better she will feel.

How she feels about herself

SPECIALTY MATERNITY STORES (BUY A GIFT CARD)

- Gap Maternity (www.gap.com)
- Old Navy Maternity (www.oldnavy.com)
- Loft Maternity (www.loft.com)
- H&M Maternity (www.HM.com)
- Forever 21 Maternity (www.Forever21.com)
- Due Maternity (www.duematernity.com/)
- Mimi Maternity (www.mimimaternity.com)
- Motherhood Maternity (www.motherhood.com)
- A Pea in the Pod (www.apeainthepod.com)
- Support local boutiques.

will determine how *you* feel. As her body changes, having something that looks good on can help make her feel more comfortable. If she thinks she looks like hell, life can be hell. If she enjoys shopping, great. If she's not a shopper, encourage her to get at least a few new things. If you have friends or families who have maternity clothes, encourage her to borrow their clothes. A friend who is done having kids is perfect.

When you find out she's pregnant or when she grows out of her prepregnancy jeans, get her a gift card to a maternity store, either a neighborhood boutique or a larger chain (she can shop online—see the sidebar on the next page). If you're going the boutique route, ask a friend of hers who has been through it for advice on where to go (and tell her to keep it a secret).

Warning: Some maternity clothes can be offensively expensive. I went shopping with my wife the other day and was blown away by the price of the jeans. I saw denim jeans for $275; I also saw some on sale for $25. Grudgingly, I admit that there is a definite difference. So when buying your gift card, walk around the store or check it out online and decide what you can afford to put on the card. Different stores have different price points. A saleswoman at one of the higher-end stores told me that the only fight she witnessed was between a husband and wife over a pair of jeans—he felt the jeans were too expensive; she didn't. One way to look at it is to amortize the jeans over a hundred days of wearing—$200 jeans would cost about $2 a day. Is $2 a day worth it to keep a pregnant woman happy? Sure (vigorously nodding my head so hard I think I pulled vertebrae).

If you're someone who likes to shop and thinks a gift card is impersonal, change your thinking. Getting the wrong size—a wrong size that's way too big—can turn you into an accidental asshole. Women don't like getting clothes ten sizes too big from the only man (other than the doctor, resident, and twenty interns) who sees her naked. Go with the gift card.

ESSENTIAL SHOPPING INFORMATION

- If you're shopping together as a couple, be careful not to be too blunt when hanging out near the dressing room. Never use the word fat—tell her it's "not flattering."

- Maternity clothing has such a short life span that return policies are often restrictive (at boutiques or department stores). *Make sure she knows the return policy before buying.* Some women like to buy clothes, take them home, try them on, and then return them (I don't know any guys who do this).
- Encourage her to ask friends or family if they can share some of their maternity clothing. It's normal to share.
- Consignment and secondhand stores can have amazing bargains. Most women only wear maternity clothes for a few months. Therefore, a lot of previously used maternity clothes can look like new.
- Do NOT buy her maternity lingerie or sexy clothing. Opt for the gift card. While you might have loving intentions, getting a piece of lingerie that's three sizes too big will turn you into an accidental asshole.
- If she decides to buy a lot of high-end clothing, she can sell the items on eBay or Craigslist when she's done. Auctions can get pretty intense for maternity jeans.

THE BOTTOM LINE:

The better she looks, the better she'll feel. The better she looks and feels, the better you'll feel.

Tip #54
THE PUSH/PREGNANCY PRESENT: A Little Something to Ease Her Pain

THE TIP:

It doesn't have to be diamonds…

> If *only* my man had known how painful it is to push a baby out of your vagina! He may have given me a push present!
>
> —*Carin, mother of one*

THE STORY:

The day I turned twenty weeks pregnant, I got home after a *long* day and found a package and card on the table with "Mommy" written on it. It was a card from my hubby and baby celebrating the fact that we were halfway through the pregnancy. The present was a wooden Willow Tree figurine called "Cherish," which is a pregnant mommy holding her tummy. Then yesterday, out of nowhere, Daddy and baby sent me a cookie bouquet (my *favorite*!)—six beautiful cookies celebrating that "It's a girl!" One of the cookies had Elizabeth's nickname on it, *Ellie*. I pretty much have the most amazing husband ever!

—*Valerie, daughter, one month*

✳✳✳

Pushing a kid out of her vagina (or having it removed from her abdomen) deserves some kind of acknowledgment. Right?

The idea of buying a new mom a special gift once she pushes the baby out isn't just made up by her. It has roots.

> I got a "pushing present"/thirtieth birthday gift. I helped pick it out—a beautiful diamond necklace.
>
> —*Heidi, mother of one, pregnant with number two*

In Europe, it's customary for women to get a gift following the birth of a child. In England, men are expected to adorn women with a beautiful ring. In India, mothers get gold and jewels for the birth. In the United States, jewelers

PUSH PRESENTS UNDER $100

- Baby charm necklaces or bracelets
- Personalized sterling silver birth necklace
- Engraved picture frame with a picture of her and her pregnant belly
- Necklace, bracelet, or earrings with the baby's birthstone
- Sleep

ENAMEL ENGRAVED BABY SHOE CHARMS
These range from the low hundreds to thousands of dollars. Do an online search for "enamel baby shoes" and you'll get a good sense of what I'm talking about. If you happen to buy online, make sure to read the return policy. She might love the idea, but not the gift.

ENGRAVED GIFTS
If you're buying something expensive but are not quite sure if she'll love it, wait until she sees it, and then engrave it. When you give it to her, tell her you wanted to wait for the birth so you could engrave the date. Once you engrave it, there is typically no returning it.

and women who want jewelry are turning this into a new gift-giving tradition.

Some guys aren't into the idea of a push present. It's not that these guys are cheap (although some might be). They say there is no greater gift than the gift of having a healthy new child, and a material thing like jewelry almost minimizes the magnitude of the event. The baby is the ultimate "push present."

So if you share this sentiment, there's nothing wrong with calling the gift something else. How about just calling it her first Mother's Day present and picking it out after the baby is born? Call it a gift from the baby and make the baby pay you back when she's old enough to work. Whatever you subscribe to, I have a hard time finding anything wrong with getting someone you love a gift that's associated with such a special event. That said, if you have a philosophical issue with the push present, explain this to your partner—just in case all her friends give her gifts, there won't be room for any misinterpretation.

A way to economize is to combine the push present with some other gift-giving occasion. It gives a "big gift" much more meaning. You can make it a surprise, or plan it as a couple's project during the last trimester. Keep in mind that shopping for jewelry allows you to say and do things you can't usually say or do. She might be too happy and distracted to be pissed off with you.

When it comes to how much to spend, it can be less than $100 or more than $1,000. Take baby bootie charms for example (charms

Month	Birthstone	Color
January	Garnet	Deep Red
February	Amethyst	Purple
March	Aquamarine	Pale Blue
April	Diamond	White, Clear
May	Emerald	Green
June	Pearl	White or Purple
July	Ruby	Red
August	Peridot, Sardonyx	Pale Green
September	Sapphire	Deep Blue
October	Opal, Pink Tourmaline	Multicolor, Pink
November	Citrine, Yellow Topaz	Yellow
December	Blue Topaz, Turquoise	Blue

are little pendants attached to a necklace or bracelet—think Monopoly pieces). Some charms cost under a hundred dollars; other charms may cost you in the thousands. One of the coolest things I've seen are little silver coinlike disks that have the baby's name engraved on them. The charms attach to a necklace/bracelet, and you can add more charms as you have more kids. If you're on a tight budget, go to a bead store with her and make something together. You can find birthstones that are extremely reasonable. If you're not sure what to get, call a maternity store and ask for advice from the manager or owner.

> I decided to give up all the food she couldn't eat, the alcohol, and other recreational habits that don't go with being pregnant.
>
> —*Mike, son, three months*

She doesn't actually have to push to get the present. Women who have C-section deliveries qualify for the push present. I couldn't imagine still having a wife or girlfriend after telling her, "It's a push present—did you push? It's not called a C-section present, is it?"

THE BOTTOM LINE:
If she wants a push present, never tell her you want a present too (unless you're wearing a protective shield around your testicles).

Tip #55
DOING THE LITTLE THINGS: And Eating, Drinking, and Behaving as If You're Pregnant

THE TIP:
The little things will have a huge impact.

THE STORY:
I do projects around the house, but the little stuff is not my area of expertise. When she was pregnant, I would focus on the small things—like not only folding her laundry, but bringing it upstairs and putting it away too. From time to time, I'd bring home a magazine she likes. Every woman has similar "small things" that she appreciates. I found the smallest things would go a long way. It's amazing how big of a reaction I could get from doing something like putting away clothes. I don't think she knew I could do it. The only problem is that now she knows I'm capable.

—*AJ, son, eighteen months*

***

Surprise her. Do something uncharacteristic—like vacuuming.

> Don't come home drunk if your wife likes to drink. Whatever she is not allowed to do during pregnancy, she does not want to hear about you doing.
>
> —*Jason, son, eight weeks*

Most men can do everything we used to do before she got pregnant. But she can't. And really, it's not fair. We can eat raw meat, drink a fifth of Jack, wear our old pants, stay out until five in the morning, hang out in smoky bars, travel, ride roller coasters, bungee jump, and ride in simulators that shake us until we vomit.

On the other hand, she's tired, uncomfortable, nauseous, and emotional. Choosing to change your lifestyle is supportive. Not eating or drinking something she can't eat or drink is compassionate. Because we don't feel the physical parts, it's easy to forget. Doing something out of the ordinary reminds us of what's coming. Housecleaning and organizing won't only help her feel supported and impress her; they will prove to be the ultimate aphrodisiac (see Tip #57).

Following are some little things you can do to help:

- Avoid eating things that she can't eat.
- Avoid alcohol, cigarettes, and illegal drugs.
- Avoid caffeinated beverages.
- Gain thirty pounds (just to show her you're totally committed).
- Gain ten pounds (just to show her you're partially committed).
- Wear an empathy belly (they actually make these things).

- Don't go out without her if she's too tired (and don't make her feel bad about it).
- Ask her what movie she wants to see instead of forcing your choice.
- Clean up around the house (a little bit goes a long way).
- Do the dishes (but load the dishwasher properly—see Tip #46).
- Cook for her. For recipes, Google "Easy (fill in the blank with name of dish you want to prepare)."
- Go shopping with her for clothes and baby stuff.
- Take a prenatal yoga class with her.
- Massage a body part of hers you don't usually touch.
- Read this book (or one of her books).
- Fold laundry (watch out for her underwear; it can have stuff).
- Take pictures of her belly and give them to her as a gift.
- Take an interest in her belly (listen to it, rub it, draw pictures on it).
- Get her a gift card or a small present.
- Get her flowers or a card.
- Listen to her when you don't usually listen.
- Allow her to win every argument.
- Do whatever the hell she asks you to do (at least for forty weeks).

THE BOTTOM LINE:

Sweep her off her feet by sweeping under her feet.

8

PREGNANT SEX

Having It, Not Having It, Fantasizing about Having It

Tip #56
PREGNANT SEX 101: The Eighteen-Inch Penis Question and More

THE TIP:
You want to get out of there right when she reaches *that* point…

THE STORY:
This is really embarrassing—but, you know how a guy has to be very adventurous when you're big and pregnant? My husband was nice enough to try to pleasure me by going down there. I didn't know that I had poor control of my

urinary tract muscles, and in the middle of the culmination, I accidentally peed in his mouth. It was a good amount of pee. He was really sweet about it—I mean *very* sweet. The whole time he was telling me that it was all right and not to worry because he

> The BEST way to seduce my pregnant wife was to give her food (I suggest bratwurst) and go masturbate to porn quickly and quietly in the other room while she ate the bratwurst.
>
> —*Doug, daughter, three, son, three*

knew that I was really so embarrassed. He just rinsed out his mouth and brushed his teeth and made sure I was okay. This tip is good advice for everyone.

—*Gloria, daughter, two*

***

No, your penis cannot poke the baby during sex.

Since you might not believe me, I asked a respected doctor with over thirty years of experience as an ob-gyn to answer this question:

QUESTION: If someone reading this has an eighteen-inch penis, would having sex hurt the baby?

ANSWER: First of all, this reader must have an enormous imagination to go along with his penis. But the rule is: if it's uncomfortable, don't do it.

He wouldn't suggest using large sex toys, but a large penis shouldn't pose a problem. Just make sure she's comfortable. He also suggests discussing any concerns with the caregiver. These questions are normal, and doctors and other care providers are comfortable addressing them. Go to a doctor's appointment and ask when your partner is out of the room (if she or you are uncomfortable asking together). You can also call your caregiver's office and talk to any of the doctors on call. Unless your doctor says "NO SEX FOR YOU!" there should be sex for you (assuming she's willing, interested, and able to have it).

> **ORAL SEX WARNING**
> If blowing air inside her vagina is your move, don't do it. This can cause an embolism and the baby and mother could die. Find another place to blow.

Assuming sex is medically safe, the idea that your penis is a few inches from your baby's head can be a bit deflating, distracting, and a total turnoff. So get that image out of your head. I know it's hard to *not* think of your penis being close to the baby because you keep reading "penis near baby," but let it go. You are *not* going to hurt the baby. The SV (sex vagina) is built for pregnant sex. As big as you might be, the baby is well protected from the outside world (your penis included). The mucous plug, the uterus (the strongest organ in the female body), and the amniotic sac are there to protect the baby. As for the fear of being grabbed by the baby, the baby is in his secure bubble. Some guys get freaked out about finishing inside; but again, it's not getting near the baby. The biggest risk of injury as a result of pregnant sex? It's her falling off the bed, knocking the wind out of you, or smacking you when you grab her nipples (see Tip #57).

> If there is zero interest on her part, you can't change it. Don't try.
>
> —Andrew, son, three, thirty-three weeks pregnant

What medical issues might shut down your sex life?

A medical condition like placenta previa (when the placenta is located on or near the cervix) or something like preterm labor, a history of miscarriages, bleeding, leaking, or a cervical condition can shut down the sex factory. If she has a normal-risk pregnancy and experiences something out of the norm like bleeding, leaking, cramping, or contracting, ask the doctor if sex can be had. And if the vagina is off-limits, there are other things you can do besides penetration.

Assuming you have clearance to enter the sex arena, appreciate that things will change. She might not be able to do what she used to do. She might fall off, roll around, feel uncomfortable, get more turned on, get less turned on, have more or less lubrication, or her body could react in ways that surprise her. She might be a different woman in the bedroom. You won't know until you get there. How to get there is addressed in Tip #57.

THE BOTTOM LINE:

The pregnant vagina can handle you. But can you handle the pregnant vagina?

Tip #57
A GUIDE TO PREGNANT SEX (VERSION 2.0): The Essentials Every Man Needs to Know

THE TIP:

1. Make her feel like you're nuts about her.
2. Always be helpful and caring.
3. Make up stuff as you go.

THE STORY:

1. I've learned that if a woman knows that you're attracted to her, she will get extremely turned on by this—even a pregnant woman. I've also learned that all women are self-conscious, especially when big and pregnant. You have to make them feel like you are crazy nuts about them all the time. Don't be timid when having sex. Do it how you used to do it. Don't change your style, or she'll interpret it as you not being as attracted or turned on. Go at it.

2. Seducing her isn't always about touching her in certain places. For example, when my wife was shellacking cabinets with a regular varnish—the kind of varnish that can give your kids three heads—I found an organic varnish that wouldn't harm the fetus. She thought it was the sweetest, most caring thing in the world. I mean, she was so happy that we had mind-blowing pregnant sex. Helping her out and showing you care is a huge turn-on.

3. The final suggestion is to make up stuff that will make her feel incredibly attractive and sexy. One time, I created an intimate moment with candles and music and told my wife that I have a secret fetish for pregnant women. I told her that I fantasize about pregnant women and visit pregnancy porn sites on the Internet. I asked her if she could indulge me just this one time. It worked one time. The next day, she realized I was full of it, but she forgave me.

—*Danny, father of four*

***

I assume you still want to have sex. Right?

To help you have the best pregnant sex, I asked expectant fathers and pregnant women from around the world to share the truth about having (or not having) pregnant sex. Before revealing the results, it's worth noting that most couples' rate of sex decreased as the pregnancy progressed. Nausea, sensitivity, medical issues, and guys getting freaked out all played a factor.

And now the results…

BEST POSITION FOR PREGNANT SEX?

- Spooning
- Woman on the side
- Doggie style (some women listed it as worst too)
- Woman on top
- Keeping it simple
- A pillow under the belly right by the pelvic bone (be careful when she starts to show or when the baby starts to move, as her pelvic area gets a bit tender)
- Woman lying in bed as usual but man underneath hips; he does all the moving (also good for post C-section)

WORST POSITION FOR PREGNANT SEX?

- Missionary—it doesn't work
- Anything requiring balance
- Anything too bouncy
- Anything involving too much flexibility

- Doggie style can be uncomfortable at times
- Woman acting as dominatrix on top (hard to carry off the stern thing when wobbling and rolling off…)
- All positions (some women are tender down there now and sex can become a turnoff)

WHAT CAN A MAN DO TO INCREASE HIS CHANCES OF HAVING SEX?

- Don't get her pregnant (most popular answer).
- Make her feel like a goddess and be experimental.
- Massage and rub her shoulders, feet…you name it.
- Run a bubble bath for her (not too hot).
- Tell her she still looks amazing, hot, and sexy.
- Make her feel important and absolutely gorgeous.
- Always think of her needs first. All else will follow.
- Do all the chores so that she has energy for sex.
- Be patient and sensual.
- Make an effort to kiss her neck and softly touch her.
- Put on some nice music, and go with the flow.
- Try kissing her and saying, "Let's have sex, hot lady."
- Help out with child number one so she's not tired and pissed off.
- Be very nice to her.
- Get her ice cream when she wants it.
- Don't ask for it (or beg for it or demand it).
- Nothing. If she doesn't want it, you'll only aggravate her by asking.
- Do not push it. (Men have no idea what it's like to be pregnant. Women already have enough demands to have you make demands.)

- Make sure she knows that she is the only one for you and that she's still attractive.
- Try sex in the morning—she's a lot less likely to be too tired.
- Masturbate…it makes you less desperate.

TIPS OR SUGGESTIONS FOR SATISFYING A PREGNANT WOMAN IN BED?

- Take more time for foreplay.
- Massage her before having sex.
- Brush your teeth. Bad breath can be a huge deal breaker when she's extra-sensitive to smells.
- Have oral sex.
- Be very gentle and avoid touching the breasts at all in the first trimester (excruciating pain doesn't usually put her in the mood).
- Let her do what she wants to do in bed (no forcing her).
- Engage in standard cuddling.
- Find out what her favorite part of her body is. (It can change when she is pregnant.) Make sure you always start by making her feel wanted and beautiful.
- Ask her what she wants you to do—her desires have probably changed and she may have very specific instructions.
- Don't be freaked out by the baby and her changing shape.
- Treat sex like a fun experimental thing rather than an inconvenience.
- Give her whatever she wants.
- Be willing to do lots of work, especially toward the end!
- Make her feel beautiful all the time.

WHAT SHOULD A MAN *NEVER* DO WITH HIS PREGNANT WIFE/PARTNER IN BED?

- Blow in her vagina—this can cause an embolism and the baby and mother can die!
- Talk about her size.
- Grab her nipples (or bite too hard).
- Tell her she's fat.
- Squeeze pressure points in her ankle which may send her into labor.
- Tell her she's too big for sex.
- Make her feel bad if there's a little blood or odor.
- Ask her if she wants anal sex or wants to give you oral sex.
- Bug her for sex or make her feel guilty for not having it.
- Watch sporting events and put moves on simultaneously.
- Assume she wants it.
- Use the words *fat* and *hormonal*.
- Say that the baby moving around is interfering too much to have sex.
- Try new things without asking first. (It's a lot easier to get hurt with a full uterus!)
- Expect her to just do anything at any time.
- Have rough sex with her (without asking first).
- Do anything she isn't up for.
- Become impatient with her.
- Put her into any position that makes her feel uncomfortable.
- Rub her belly and say "Wow" like you can't believe she's *that* enormous.
- Get upset if something leaks or squirts.

MOST HILARIOUS OR AWKWARD SEX MOMENT?

- "I farted."
- "It was a month and a half before our due date and while we were fooling around, he stopped me and asked why I was drooling all over his chest. I wasn't; I was lactating!"
- "I would want it more than he did. He couldn't keep up with me."
- "The baby kicked while in missionary. My fiancé could feel her kick him too."
- "I had an overall lack of coordination as the pregnancy progressed—we had klutzy lovemaking."
- "When I was pregnant with my second, I was huge and knocked the wind out of him with my belly."
- "The baby started moving during the deed—we kept going, though."
- "I was sick at the sight and smell of his semen."
- "I got leg cramps in the middle of it."
- "The baby would use my cervix as a trampoline and he would enter at the same time."
- "As I was trying to get comfy near the end, I rolled off a few times."
- "I wasn't able to move when I was about thirty-eight weeks pregnant. I was huge and there was not too much I could do from my end."
- "I would wake up extremely horny. I practically jumped on him. This is a big deal as I have *never* been a morning sex person."
- "I peed in his mouth."

THE BOTTOM LINE:

You never knew how much you loved having sex with a pregnant woman…

Tip #58
MEN WHO DON'T WANT SEX: If You're Rejecting Your Pregnant Partner

THE TIP:

If you don't want sex with her while she's pregnant, make sure to help her feel beautiful and desirable.

THE STORY:

We had a lot of sex at the beginning of the pregnancy. As the months progressed, the sex slowed down. During the last couple of months, he no longer wanted it at all. I know it was awkward for him (I once got a leg cramp in the middle of it) and that he was concerned for the baby, but his lack of interest made me feel ugly and bad about myself. Even if he didn't want to have sex, it would have been nice if he found other ways to make me feel attractive and loved. It didn't have to be a sexual thing; he could have planned something like a romantic dinner for no reason just to show me he still cared.

—*Lesha, sons, eight months and two and a half*

✳✳✳

Some men don't want to have sex with a pregnant woman. They just can't do it.

It's one of the phenomena of being an expectant father. It might be a fear of hurting the baby. It might be your partner's physical appearance. (Women don't want to hear this, but it can happen.) The huge changes, long hours working to get ready for the arrival, or mounting anxiety might shut down your sex drive. If you don't want it and your partner does, be sensitive to how this is interpreted in her world.

Pregnant woman are not especially good with rejection. In general, no one loves rejection. And a woman who is uncomfortable in her Expectant Mother Thong (see Tip #42: The Hormonal Pregnant Woman) is especially vulnerable. She sees rejection as something being wrong with her. She sees you as not being attracted to her. She sees you as being detached and uninterested. It's more than the sex.

If you're not interested in sex, try something different. You can touch, kiss, or rub. If you're still not in the mood, it's crucial for you to explain the circumstances behind the sexual rejection. If it's too sensitive to share with her or if you're not sure why you feel this way, just tell her it makes you uncomfortable, but it has nothing to do with her not being beautiful. Blame it on being weirded out by having a baby so close to your penis. Whatever you do, just make a big effort to stay physically connected and show her that you still love her. Hug her more, kiss her more, rub her down more, get her flowers or a gift—do something so

> We used to have sex every day before I got pregnant. Since I got pregnant, it's been gradually less and less. I'm starting to feel resentful toward him because I have needs too. It took two to make this baby, and he still wants me to pleasure him.
> —Claire, thirty-seven weeks pregnant

that she will never doubt how much you love her and care about her.

NO SEX WARNING

If you find that you're not as physically attracted to your pregnant partner, recognize that this may have nothing to do with her body. Yes, there are physical changes, but on some level, her new look is a constant reminder of a lifetime of responsibility and huge changes coming your way. (By the way, they're great changes.) That's one reason some guys freak out and distance themselves (emotionally or physically).

> **ATTENTION, REJECTED EXPECTANT FATHERS**
>
> If your partner is the one who doesn't want sex with you, revisit Tip #16: The Rejected Expectant Father. Also consider discussing the suggestions in Tip #57 with her. This might help you figure out how to seduce her and get her in the mood.

If you can't give it up, don't give up on loving her. Do other things to reassure her that you're still into her. Find other ways to please her. I guarantee that at some point during the pregnancy (or your life), she's done it for you.

THE BOTTOM LINE:

If possible, let her have sex with you. She's done it for you.

Tip #59
MEN WHO HAVE SEX ALONE: How Pregnant Women Feel about Porn

THE TIP:

Some pregnant women don't like it when men look at attractive naked or half-naked women who aren't pregnant. Don't argue.

THE STORY:

A neighbor gave me some magazines and left an *FHM* magazine for my husband, which I put straight into the garbage bin. (I used to look like the girls in those magazines, but I obviously looked nothing like that anymore!) Anyway, I told him that the neighbor gave me some magazines, but I threw the *FHM* away. He then went on to ask me why I tossed it and argued with me because he never goes out of his way to buy these kinds of magazines for himself and would have liked to flip through it! I stormed off in a huff because I honestly felt threatened and jealous. Here I am, carrying his baby, and he doesn't want to make love to me at all, but it's okay for him to look at girls in expensive underwear that I could never wear because I'm having his baby!

—*Claire, thirty-seven weeks pregnant*

***

> My wife knows that I have the propensity to look at porn online—she gives me that. She just looks at me and rolls her eyes. We used to watch it together so she understands.
>
> —*Loving Porn-Consuming Husband*

> Pregnant sex for me was like I was back in high school again. The sex was great but lonely. Again, Internet porn, some lotion, tissues, and ten minutes. On occasion, my wife would consider it foreplay when she cued up PornHub for me on the computer and told me to come to bed when I'm done.
>
> —*Doug, daughter, three, son, three*

Don't get caught with porn if she's not cool with porn.

Some pregnant women encourage their partners to use porn—it gives them a break. Others find it disgusting and off-limits. If your partner has a problem with porn and she's not interested in sex, that's a problem.

The idea of you looking at another woman and getting turned on is hard to explain if you get caught (especially if you're not having sex with your pregnant partner). Whether it's a men's magazine or a hard-core website, when it comes to focusing your sexual energy elsewhere, it's impossible to convince the love of your life that porn is a harmless outlet that has nothing to do with your level of attraction to her. By definition, if she's harmed, it's not harmless.

Some women (pregnant or not) feel threatened and violated by porn. They question their marriage, they question the relationship, and they question themselves. And pregnant women can be especially uncomfortable with porn. Even if you're into pregnant porn, it's hard to explain. And I know—you've been using it your entire life and you love your partner, but she's harder to convince. As a rule:

1. Do not get caught.
2. If caught, apologize and explain that you love her.
3. Use your imagination.

If your antiporn pregnant partner catches you using porn, expect her to be upset, doubt your level of attraction to her, and feel betrayed. She might think you're cheating. She might yell, cry, or just leave you (yes, it happens). Most women (pregnant or not) don't understand that porn and masturbation can be an outlet for stress and anxiety—they see it as a threat or reflection of your lack of satisfaction or commitment.

What women may not realize is that some guys have been consuming porn and masturbating long before marriage. This doesn't make it okay, but the point is that it's habitual and can have little to do with his level of commitment or desire for his partner. Sure, there are healthier ways to relieve stress, but women aren't as threatened by a guy participating in a fantasy bowling league as opposed to a guy watching fantasy bowling porn. (I might find that a little strange too.)

Should you have to explain the unexplainable, tell your partner that this is more about stress and anxiety than the images on the screen. If she can't get over it, get counseling together. Make sure she knows you love her, and don't give her more reasons to doubt your commitment. If you want to stop using but can't, or if she wants to you to stop but you can't, seek support and treatment. While you might think porn is harmless, the moment it causes harm, it stops being harmless.

THE BOTTOM LINE:

Getting caught watching pregnant porn doesn't make it any better…

SHOPPING FOR BABY

Something So Little Needs So Much

SHOPPING FOR BABY: How Could Something So Little
Need So Much?

THE TIP:
Go to the store and register so when people want to get
something for you, they'll know what to buy.

THE STORY:
A lot of people are willing to help out, but they don't know
what to get us. We're having a shower soon, so we are in
the process of registering. It's overwhelming how much
stuff there is online. I find it helps to see it and touch it.

This weekend, I spent over four hours shopping—two at Walmart and two and a half at Babies "R" Us. We were pre-registering—and no, this isn't registering; it's what happens *before* you register. I have never felt more lost and overwhelmed in four aisles of a store. Do we need this? Which bottles are the right bottles? She looks at me like, "I don't know which ones to get." And I'm thinking the same thing. Another suggestion is to pack a snack and water—you don't want to have a hungry pregnant wife on your hands.

—*Scott, six months pregnant*

> Going to Babies "R" Us for a woman is like going to Best Buy for a man.
>
> —*Cathy, sons, four months and three and a half*

***

Welcome to the baby superstore. Let me show you around.

Here you will find the: *strollers, car seats, infant seats, cribs, bassinettes, co-sleepers, monitors, baby carriers, diapers, diaper bags, diaper dispensers, diaper rash creams, baby wipes, changing pads, changing tables, baby furniture sets, rockers, pacifiers, bottles, nipples, blankets, swaddlers, lotions, rectal thermometers, swings, bedding sets, layettes (the baby's first clothing, bedding, and essentials for the first three months), hats, socks, shoes, towels, washcloths, baby bathtubs, baby soaps, bathtub toys, rubbing alcohols, cotton balls (to clean the belly button), antigas medications, nasal aspirators, infant medicines, infant nail clippers, hairbrushes, combs, tweezers, brushes to clean bottles,*

> My wife hates to shop. We only order things online.
>
> —*Todd, son, four months*

Video monitors are worth every single penny.

—Jon, son, three, thirty-three weeks pregnant

toys, stuffed animals, rattles, bouncy seats, kids' CDs, breast milk storage bottles (if nursing), breast pumps, and much, much more!

It can be overwhelming. So here are some tips to keep in mind while buying things for baby:

- First locate the gliders/rocking chairs. They are a great place to sit while she shops (if you're not a shopper).
- Find something that interests you so you don't go out of your mind (focus on the stroller, baby gates, or a construction project).
- Bring food in case she gets hungry (but don't eat it all first).
- Shop at the houses of friends and family. We borrowed a stroller, a co-sleeper, baby carrier, baby clothing, maternity clothes, and stuff they didn't even know we took (only kidding, we asked).
- Don't open new stuff you purchase until you need it (this way you can still return it).
- *Save all receipts* (you'll need them if you break something during assembly).
- Know the return policy. Some stores have limited windows because babies outgrow stuff so fast.
- Get storage containers (great for holding all the little things).
- Let an expert assemble

Just get everything from Amazon. You don't need to be running around. And she doesn't either.

—Jim, daughter, two, son, eleven

REQUIRED READING

Baby Bargains by Denise and Alan Fields. This *amazing* book will answer most of your questions. Sign up for their newsletter and get alerts on recalls or products mentioned in the book. The book hits on all the major purchases and offers pros, cons, and inside information on the most essential products (www.babybargains.com).

the crib unless you're a handyman (build this into the cost when budgeting).

- Always ask if there's a coupon when checking out. (Sometimes a sales-clerk will pull one out of thin air.)
- Use your smartphone to search online for coupons. A lot of stores will scan the coupon on your phone and may even have apps for this purpose.
- If people buy gifts you won't use for several months, consider returning them for store credit. Buy an item when you need it.
- Kids outgrow expensive clothes as fast as inexpensive clothes.
- Shopping with grandparents can be cost-effective.
- Don't buy the big-ticket items right away (cowork-ers might pool their money and buy you a ridiculous stroller).
- Buy the essentials and wait to get everything else as you need it.
- Take advantage of free shipping and bulk discounts when ordering online.
- Have the heavy stuff shipped to your door (diapers, for-mula, big-ticket items).

- Expensive bedding will get burped on, peed on, and pooped on.
- Babies don't care about thread count.
- If you're putting together a crib, car seat, or anything that swings, moves, makes noise, or needs batteries, *read the directions first* (this one is hard).
- Over time, all diaper dispenser systems will smell like a Porta-Potty on a hot summer's day.
- Register everything you buy with the manufacturer so that you will receive recall messages or other essential information.
- If getting things secondhand, make sure they're safe. (Never buy a used car seat or a crib that has a history that can't be verified.) Check the recall list by visiting www.recalls.gov.
- Car seats expire (crazy, I know).

WARNING

If you borrow or buy something used on Craigslist or eBay, make sure it's still safe. Government safety guidelines are constantly changing. For the latest info, visit www.CPSC.gov (Consumer Product Safety Commission).

RECENT CHANGE REGARDING CRIB SAFETY

Beginning June 28, 2011, all cribs manufactured and sold (including resale) must comply with new and improved federal safety standards. The new rules, which apply to full-size and non-full-size cribs, prohibit the manufacture or sale of traditional drop-side rail cribs, strengthen crib slats and mattress supports, improve the quality of hardware, and require more rigorous testing. The details of the rule are available on CPSC's website at www.cpsc.gov /businfo/frnotices/fr11/cribfinal.pdf.

THE BOTTOM LINE:

It's mind-boggling how someone under ten pounds can need so much.

Tip #61
THE EMOTIONAL PURCHASE: You'll Cry When You See the Bill

THE TIP:

As a rule, avoid making emotional purchases (with a few exceptions).

THE STORY:

My wife has always been an emotional shopper. There were several times when she wanted to make an emotional purchase for the baby. One incident that sticks out was a $2,000 bassinet—something that would last only a couple months. Even the less expensive bassinet was $500. We avoided that purchase altogether. It's not tough for me to say "No." I figure if I'm having a baby girl, I need to get used to saying it! If you think your wife can spend, your wife and daughter combined can spend enough to bankrupt you. If there is a practical use for something, a "no" can turn into a "yes." It's the difference between what we *want* and what we *need*. From time to time, we do indulge in the wants. When she was pregnant, she wanted a piece of jewelry that represented the circle of life, so after our daughter was born, she "bought" it and presented the jewelry to her mom. Buying the stroller was an exercise in wearing me down. It was like the movie *Groundhog Day*—over and over and over again

> Watch her like a hawk; salespeople know how easy it is to sell expensive bedding to a pregnant lady. They can convince you to buy a lot of things that you don't know whether you'll need yet.
>
> —*Emily, mother of two*

until we finally got the one I swore we would never get. My wife jokes that I'm the meanest man on the planet. My motto: take care of the pennies and the pounds take care of themselves.

—*Kevin, daughter, three months*

> Talk to people who have done it before you. There will be tons of stuff that you don't need for the health, happiness, and safety of your new baby. I felt that some advertising and sales tactics try to prey on your desire to do what's best for your new baby.
>
> —*Brian, daughter, one*

***

If you are on a budget, shopping for the baby can be an emotional experience. Seeing the credit card statement will make most men break down in tears. There's a lot to buy and emotions are tied to them all (even a rectal thermometer). From the bedding to the crib to the stroller to the car seat—if you're not careful, you can easily spend a small fortune.

Often it's the man who ends up playing the role of the bad guy. Here's the problem: she's physically and emotionally transformed and busy spending all her time researching a purchase. When she's ready to pull the trigger, in walks the guy complaining that it costs too much or that *Consumer Reports* says it's the wrong choice. Then it can become a fight. And when it comes to fighting with a pregnant woman, even if you win, you have lost.

Some strategies to prevent her from getting sad and you feeling bad:

- Figure out what you need versus what you want. Create a list. NEEDS on one side, WANTS on the other side.

Stick to what you need and wait to see if you can get what you want as a gift. The emotional purchase can wait.

- Set a budget early, figure out what you can afford, and then find a way to stick to it. If you have a budget in place, you can refer to it when her emotions (or yours) run high. Blame it on the budget.
- Be involved early on in the process. This means having a sense of what things cost and why they cost that much. For example, not all strollers are created equal. The more expensive strollers might last longer than the less expensive ones. The price doesn't tell the entire story.
- When it comes to *great* deals, make sure the company can deliver and that what they're delivering is safe. Since we had our first baby, I've watched one baby furniture store chain go out of business and another change owners. One company would take orders and *never* deliver the cribs. Investigate their customer service policies before making the purchase (do an online search and post comments in new parent community forums).
- Wait to buy stuff. Once the baby is born, you'll really know what you need as opposed to what you think you'll need.

THE BOTTOM LINE:

The emotional purchase cry-fecta (like a trifecta):

1. The salesperson cries from joy because her commission is so huge.
2. Your pregnant partner cries from joy because the nursery is so beautiful.
3. You cry because you have to donate a limb to pay for it all.

THE TIP:

All strollers break down differently. Once you figure out how to make one collapse, help out your fellow man.

THE STORY:

Shopping for the stroller was one of the most memorable experiences. You walk down the aisle and see a row of guys struggling with the strollers trying to collapse them, but no two collapse the same way. You see some guys just standing there staring blankly at the stroller. Meanwhile other guys are kicking, struggling, pushing, and pulling until the strollers break down or just break. There are so many different levers and buttons. Once I figured out how to collapse a stroller, I would walk down the aisle and help out other guys struggling with them. How a stroller collapses was a factor in what we decided to buy. We ended up with two strollers. We went with the smallest stroller that fit in my trunk and a jogging stroller for home. Honestly, we still can't figure out how to break down the jogging stroller.

—*Chris, son, twenty-two months*

***

Things to keep in mind: make sure he can use it. Can he figure out how to open it and close it? Is he too tall to reach the handles? Make sure it can take a beating. Strollers get bashed around a lot.

—*Emily, mother of two*

> The biggest purchase for me was the stroller. I didn't care about cost. I wanted something that was going to hold up, I could use for running, was city-appropriate, and easy. We did the Valco Tri Mode and it was awesome.
>
> —*Moss, daughters,*
> *three and five*

The 1800s marked the industrial revolution. The 2000s marked the stroller revolution. Top engineering, research and development, and state-of-the-art materials have thrust us into the future. It's the golden age of strollers.

Strollers vary in function, style, and price. You can get an umbrella stroller for $10 or a fancy stroller for over $1,000. The perfect stroller is like the perfect pair of jeans—it's a personal choice based on a list of very specific criteria. There are real differences between the most inexpensive and the most expensive ones. Adjustable versus nonadjustable handles, plastic versus rubber wheels, storage capacity, weight, and versatility are some things to consider.

When you walk into the stroller showroom, it's important to arrive with a budget, specific needs, and suggestions of like-minded friends. Bring the *Baby Bargains* book or a *Consumer Reports* with you. Without a budget and guidelines in mind, it's like walking into a car dealership that sells Mercedes and Ford Escorts on the same lot. The emotions of imagining a ride with your new baby can push you into buying a stroller that's beyond your needs or means. Some things to keep in mind when shopping:

- Know your budget. (Again, discuss this with each other before setting foot in the store.)

- Is the stroller safe and durable? (Check out the *Baby Bargains* book.)
- How does it feel during test driving? (Put something in it that weighs the same as a baby to get the feel for turning, braking, and acceleration.)
- Do you kick the wheels while strolling? (Some guys are taller than their partners.)
- Do you have to bend over to push it? (That will kill your back over time.)
- Does it hurt your back, shoulders, or extremities to push? (Adjustable arms can be helpful.)
- How much space is in the cargo area beneath the basket? (If there isn't room to hold the bag, you'll be holding the bag.)
- Are you going to be off-roading or mostly mall strolling? (Sidewalks cause wear and tear.)
- Is it easy to clean and machine-washable? (Spilled milk can stink. I have to wash ours once every couple of months.)
- Is the size right? (Some strollers are too wide for store aisles, not unlike Hummers on the road.)
- Which direction will the baby face?
- Will the stroller grow as your baby grows?
- What matters most to you (or her)—vanity or functionality?

Let me be the one to break the news. You'll want more than one stroller. Why? One will be lightweight to keep in the trunk. The other will be bigger and heavier for longer walks. One thing that I wish I knew during our first pregnancy—our big stroller didn't have an option for an infant to sit facing us. I think looking at her would have cost us another $400. So instead, we carried a picture of her and looked at it while we strolled.

MY INTERVIEW WITH A STROLLER EXPERT

QUESTION: What is the biggest mistake men make when shopping for strollers?

ANSWER: Expectant fathers often downplay how often they will be using the stroller and defer to their wives, thinking that the stroller should better suit her. But a six-foot-four father and a four-foot-eleven mother cannot comfortably use the same stroller unless the handlebar adjusts for user height.

QUESTION: Your tips for shopping for a stroller on a budget?

ANSWER: Always consider your current needs and

how they might change with the addition of a child. Ask yourself where you will be using the stroller most often, as terrain determines wheel type, which will affect the weight of the stroller. If you jog, ask yourself if you will continue to jog after the baby is born and if you will be in the market for a jogging stroller. Also take into account your body type versus your wife's body type and the height factor. If you are on a budget, buy one or two quality aluminum-framed strollers (one for rough terrain or jogging and one to travel with) instead of buying a cheap plastic stroller, which will likely need to be replaced after very little real use.

QUESTION: Tips for shopping with a limitless budget?

ANSWER: If you have a limitless budget, treat yourself to something top of the line and make your partner happy. That said, limit yourself to two or three good strollers per child unless you also have limitless storage space. (**Author's note:** Not sure if I agree with this one.)

QUESTION: Ever seen a couple get in a fight while shopping?

ANSWER: Yes, although I can't recall any specific details. Often, if the husband appears to be apathetic or bummed because he's missing the game, his wife will pick up on it. On the flip side, his wife should be concerned with more than just the color or brand name of the stroller and take into account her husband's concerns about mechanics and warranty.

QUESTION: Any essentials that guys shopping with their pregnant partners should keep in mind?

ANSWER: Guys need to remain logical and focused, as their pregnant partners are often emotional time bombs.

THE BOTTOM LINE:

Safety, comfort (yours, hers, and baby's), warranty, and price do matter. If opting for a less stylish stroller, consider aftermarket rims, a subwoofer, and a rear spoiler.

Tip #63
THE CRIB, FURNITURE, AND NURSERY: No Assembly Required...If You Pay Them to Assemble It

THE TIP:
Test it before you allow your wife and baby to use it.

THE STORY:
I've always wanted an old-fashioned rocking chair—not one of those padded gliders, but a real rocking chair. As a gift, my husband surprised me by getting the rocking chair I had always wanted. It was one of those chairs that he was supposed to construct. He put it together and had it all ready for me. The first night home, when the baby got up in the middle of the night, I picked her up and walked over to the chair to feed her. The rocking chair was gorgeous. I went to sit in the chair, and all of a sudden, I fell flat on the floor. I fell down hard and fast and screamed as loud as I could scream. I broke my fall with my shoulder so I wouldn't

drop my daughter. There was wood everywhere—I'm not kidding, it was straight out of a cartoon. That was the last thing he ever built. I would never trust a changing table he constructed.

—Rebekah, daughters, two and four

***

The baby's room will need a crib, furniture, a rocker (or glider), a changing table, and a 42-inch flat screen TV. (Just kidding…it will need a 52-inch flat screen TV.)

When shopping remember TCS—Timing, Cost, and Safety.

There are two timing issues. The first is the time it takes from the date you order furniture until it's delivered (it can be months). So when she suggests shopping for baby at week thirteen, she's not just being overexcited. She's making sure you get everything in time. The second time issue is that when a pregnant woman's nesting instinct kicks in, she's going to want it done when she wants it done—unless you come up with a timeline before her nesting instincts kick in (see Tip #48), she will be relentless. Create a timeline for when you'll get things done before she brings it up.

When it comes to the cost, you can spend hundreds or thousands. You can get new furniture, used furniture, pre-assembled furniture, or furniture you need to assemble. If you're thinking of buying used furniture, make sure it's safe (check for recalls—see the sidebar). If you purchase furniture that needs to be assembled, my best advice is to pay a professional to do it (the delivery person should be trained). If it costs you $50 to make sure it's done correctly, it's a small price to pay for safety. There's no room for errors (or extra pieces) when it comes to your baby's safety. If you assemble the crib, have pictures of what the finished product is supposed to look like. Check out the furniture on the showroom floor. Take digital photos from all angles (underneath too). Even if there's a picture on the box, it's worth making sure you have some kind of visual guide to go along with the 1,421 assembly steps. If you find that you have extra pieces, don't just toss them aside. Call a professional.

THE TOP FIVE HIDDEN HOME HAZARDS

1. Magnets: since 2005, there have been one death, eight injuries, and eight million toys recalled due to magnets.
2. Recalled products: each year there are about four hundred recalls. Get dangerous products out of the home. Join the U.S. Consumer Product Safety Commission's "Drive to One Million" campaign and sign up for free email notifications at www.cpsc.gov/cpsclist.aspx. An email from CPSC is not spam—it could save a life.
3. Tip-overs (e.g., furniture, shelves, chairs, etc.): average of twenty-two deaths per year; in 2006, thirty-one deaths and an estimated three thousand injuries. Anchor your furniture to the wall or consult an expert.

THE TOP FIVE HIDDEN HOME HAZARDS (cont.)

4. Windows and coverings: average of twelve deaths annually from window cords; average of nine deaths and an estimated 3,700 injuries to children annually from window falls.

5. Pool and spa drains (the suction can pull small children down): fifteen injuries, two fatalities between 2002 and 2004.

(Source: U.S. Consumer Product Safety Commission, 2007)

When budgeting for the nursery, there are ways to spend less and still create a cool space—things like adding a wallpaper border, stenciling names with paint, printing out photos of animals and framing them, photographing the baby's body parts, or using a quilt that comes with the bedding as a wall hanging. (Quilts shouldn't be in the crib with the newborn anyway.) Before buying something, see if it can be made. If you're decorating a room before you know the baby's gender, you can use neutral colors and add gender-specific wallpaper borders, stencils, wall hangings, etc., after the baby arrives.

As for safety, contact a baby-proofing service and have an expert walk through your place and point out problem areas. Make sure you have a carbon monoxide detector and fire alarm inside the baby's room. If the bedroom is on a high floor, consider an escape ladder. If there are window coverings, make sure there are no strangulation hazards. Before the baby starts crawling, make sure you cover up or remove doorstops (the rubber pieces on the end can be choking hazards), cover exposed outlets, baby-proof sliding drawers, install baby gates, lower the temperature on the hot water tank, and anchor anything to the wall that can tip over and fall. When it comes to crib safety, take note of the following suggestions from the U.S. Consumer Product Safety Commission (CPSC).

For cribs there should be:

- A firm, tight-fitting mattress so a baby cannot get trapped between the mattress and the crib.
- No missing, loose, broken, or improperly installed screws, brackets, or other hardware on the crib or mattress support.
- No more than 2⅜ inches (about the width of a soda can) between crib slats so a baby's body cannot fit through the slats; no missing or cracked slats.
- No corner posts over 1/16 inch high, so a baby's clothing cannot catch.
- No cutouts in the headboard or footboard so a baby's head cannot get trapped.

For mesh-sided cribs or playpens, look for:

- Mesh less than ¼ inch in size, smaller than the tiny buttons on a baby's clothing.
- Mesh with no tears, holes, or loose threads that could entangle a baby.

- Mesh securely attached to top rail and floor plate.
- Top rail cover with no tears or holes.
- If staples are used, they are not missing, loose, or exposed.

BEFORE BUYING OR BORROWING A CRIB, READ THIS ALERT
Q & A FROM THE CPSC WEBSITE

How do I know whether the specific crib that I own/use in my child care facility meets the new standards? You cannot tell from looking at a crib whether it meets the new standards. It is not likely that cribs in use before the Commission issued its crib rule in December 2010 will comply with the new standards. If you are considering purchasing new cribs that meet the standards, you may want to ask the manufacturer or retailer whether the crib complies with 16 CFR 1219 (the new standard for full-size cribs) or 16 CFR 1220 (the new standard for non-full-size cribs). Manufacturers are required to test samples of their cribs to the new standards and to certify that they comply with the new standards. They must provide this certification to the retailer.

(Source: www.cpsc.gov/onsafety/2011/06/the-new-crib-standard-questions-and-answers)

THE BOTTOM LINE:

When assembling things, leftover pieces are a sign that you shouldn't be assembling things. Hire a pro and sleep easy knowing everything is safe.

Tip #64
THE CAR SEAT(S): You'll Probably Need Two (I Know, It's Ridiculous)

THE TIP:

This might be the first time you read installation directions from cover to cover. It might also be the first time you'll realize your backseat has a LATCH system.

THE STORY:

From the moment I found out we were expecting to the moment I took the infant car seat out of the box, I was adjusting to the idea of parenthood. Installing the car seat was the first time I felt like I was being a dad. I had a distinct feeling of fatherly responsibility—that I was helping this little person to be safe. After removing the seat from the box, I studied it and read the manual from cover to cover. I must have read every single word, although I did skip the German and French parts. There are a couple of different ways to install the car seat. There's the seat belt installation and then there's the LATCH installation. I was relieved to find out that we had the LATCH system (didn't even know it when I got the car, just got lucky). I highly recommend the LATCH system. Once the seat was firmly in place, I practiced with a teddy bear that I estimated to

CAR SEAT ESSENTIALS

- Install the car seat early and practice before getting to the hospital.
- Get it checked at a child seat fitting station (www.safercar.gov/parents/carseats.htm).
- Look for sales during the months leading up to the due date.
- Register your seat with the manufacturer.
- If your seat is in a serious car accident, replace it.
- The life span of a car seat can be five years or fewer (then replace it).

be the same size as a baby to get a feel for the straps and buckles. I'll never forget the image of this little teddy bear strapped in the seat with a five-point harness, ready to go for a ride.
—*Josh, son, thirteen months*

***

I own five car seats. When we found out that we were having a third baby, we had to get rid of the old car seats and buy narrower ones. When my kids were infants, we opted for an infant seat with two bases (one for each car). Once they outgrew the infant seat, we moved them to convertible car seats. We also chose to keep our kids rear-facing as long as possible. Some people like to turn their kids around, but it's safest to keep them rear-facing.

Know your options. Read the instructions. Get involved in this purchase. Start by picking up the book *Baby Bargains* by Denise and Alan Fields. This is the ultimate guide to help you figure out what you need and don't need. You'll figure out if you want an infant seat or a convertible car seat (this seat "converts" from rear-facing to front-facing). You might find a seat that can grow with your child, but don't plan on it.

When it comes to installing your infant car seat, read the directions and practice a good month before the due date (much better than in the hospital parking lot the morning you drive home). And honestly, it takes practice. When it comes to the physical installation, even if you read the manual in every language, get it checked at a child seat fitting station. I was shocked to discover that I did it wrong. Considering that roughly 80 percent of child safety seats are *not* installed properly, installing it early will give you time to get it checked out. You can find fitting locations via the National Highway Traffic Safety Administration (NHTSA) website www.SaferCar.org. Select the "Locate a Child Seat Fitting Station" box on the page, and it will direct you. You can also call your local fire department or police station and ask where to find a child seat fitting station.

LIKE BREAST MILK, CAR SEATS EXPIRE TOO

Yes, it's true. Car seats don't stay safe forever. If you are using a car seat from a friend or family, check with the manufacturer to see if it's still safe. We just had to replace my daughter's seat after six years.

For the most updated info on car seats, visit: www.safercar.gov /parents/carseats.htm.

CAR SEAT SUGGESTION

Check your car owner's manual and see if you have a LATCH system. Most newer cars have one (it just makes it easier to install the seat or the base). Having a LATCH system means that instead of using the seat belts in the car, you're able to use the latches and belts on the actual car seat. It's a lot easier and faster.

When it comes to cost, look for sales and coupons. You won't need a convertible seat for several months, so try to find a bargain. Never buy a used car seat or a seat with a history that can't be verified. (You don't want a seat that's been in a car accident, as seats in serious car accidents should be discarded.) When it comes to cutting costs, the car seat isn't the place do it. Our infant seat was our most used baby item during the first few months. We took it absolutely everywhere. In the earliest weeks, we even used the infant seat inside the crib. Our daughter slept better on an incline, and the seat was the most comfortable place for her.

When it comes to the styles, makes, and models, look them up in the *Baby Bargains* book (and no, I get no commission for promoting this; it's just an awesome resource). The book covers the high, middle, and lower tiers of the most common brands. The NHTSA website (www.nhtsa.gov) also provides safety information, ease-of-use information, the latest recalls, and other vital information. And when you buy your seat, make sure you register it at the manufacturer's website. (Include your email address when registering so you'll have a better chance of being informed if there's a recall or another issue that comes up.) I think that covers the car seat.

THE BOTTOM LINE:

You will install the car seat wrong. I was so sure I did it right, but I didn't. Get it checked by a pro. Visit: www.SaferCar.org

Looking for more great features to help you prep for your new arrival? Get the *Dad's Expecting Too* week-by-week pregnancy tracker, designed for dads and their partners, along with weekly updates about baby, your partner, and you at DadsExpectingToo.com.

✳✳✳

To get the latest news, info, facts, and stats for new and expecting parents, follow @DadsExpecting on Twitter and check out the Dad's Expecting Facebook Page at www.Facebook.com /DadsExpecting.

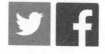

10

PASSING THE TIME

Things to Do During the Second and Third Trimesters

Tip #65
THE BABY'S SEX: To Peek or Not to Peek, That Is the Question

THE TIP:
That one moment of pure surprise will be a memory that will stay with you forever.

THE STORY:
We did not find out the gender of our baby. But we both were confident that the baby was a boy. About a month from my wife's due date, I became convinced that the baby was actually a girl. There was no particular reason—it was

just an intense gut feeling. When my wife went into the hospital to deliver, we told the nurses that I was going to stay "up north" to support my wife, but that I wanted to be the one to announce to my wife whether the baby was a boy or girl. As it turned out, things didn't go quite according to plan, and my wife ended up with a C-section. Surprisingly, the doctor still invited me to look over the sterile curtain at one point to announce the baby's gender. To this day, I remember my thought process: I saw the little head come out, then the shoulders, and then the beautiful belly. I remember thinking how perfect the baby girl was. Then the baby's waist emerged, and I remember thinking, "Oh my god, she has a scrotum." Then it dawned on me that the baby was a boy, not a girl, as I'd inexplicably expected.

—*Jon, son, three, thirty-three weeks pregnant*

BONUS STORY:

We waited to find out. I think it's the only way to go with the first child. (We don't have a second yet, but we'll probably find out for number two, maybe not if I have any say in the matter.) The true surprise of the moment is amazing. As a dad, you have a front row seat to "the show," and you are the first to know. You then get to tell your wife, one of the only times you will actually know more about your child than she does. And then comes the fun part—going into the waiting room to tell the grandparents. The

> Never waited. Always found out. It helped us plan and made it "real-er" somehow. It helps to kind of envision things and makes the wait more bearable (for her anyway).
>
> —*Patrick, expecting number six—a girl*

> We waited for several reasons: (1) we love surprises, (2) we believe in delayed gratification, and (3) we thought it was odd when some of our friends found out the sex of their unborn child, named it, and started addressing it as a real person.
>
> —Mike, son, three months

look on their faces is priceless. At that point, you feel like the most important person in the world. A lot of people like to know the sex so they can "set up" everything before the baby comes home, but it's really not an issue. I wouldn't paint the room pink, but a nice light blue or yellow works for either sex. Everything else can wait until after he/she is born. That moment of surprise will stay with me forever.

—*AJ, son, eighteen months*

***

We waited. We waited again. And we are waiting one more time. Here's how we see it—there are so few happy surprises in life that are this amazing. There's nothing like that moment of discovering the sex. It's the ultimate BIG reveal.

All it takes is an over-the-counter test that uses her urine to determine the sex. You can also find out via ultrasound as early as week twelve.

For us, not knowing and guessing was a great distraction (but also annoying at times). Most of our family and friends swore it was a boy. My wife swore it was a girl. I just swore. I studied the twenty-week ultrasound meticulously looking for a penis. I was convinced I saw a penis, but I later discovered the suspected penis was actually a foot (I was so proud of that big foot for months). We were subjected to lunar charts, the needle/ring on the thread test (if the ring

FLIP A COIN, BOY OR GIRL?

Medical Methods to Determine Gender: ultrasound (assuming the baby exposes him- or herself), amniocentesis (for high-risk pregnancies), and CVS testing (for high-risk pregnancies).

Old Wives' Tales to Determine Gender: baby's heart rate under 140 = boy, over 140 = girl. Carrying low = boy, carrying high = girl. No morning sickness in the first trimester = boy. Right boob bigger than the other = boy, bigger left boob = girl. Clear urine = girl (bright yellow urine that glows in the dark = you need to drink more water). Flipping a coin: heads = boy, tails = girl (actually, I just made the coin one up).

swings in a circle, it's a girl; if it moves like a pendulum, it's a boy), and constant questions about her food cravings (as if that would indicate the sex). How my wife was carrying the baby was also the topic of a lot of discussion. The family thought because she was carrying low it had to be a boy (she's not that tall, so anything she carries is low).

Shopping for the baby meant picking out both boy clothes and girl clothes—considering that she likes shopping, this just gave her that much more to do. The stores don't make you buy a lot of these things until you need them. She had two boxes waiting for her once the baby was born. When it came to the nursery, we picked a neutral color and used a wallpaper border that matched the bedding. Whatever the sex, we were ready.

The majority of people I know find out. A lot of times, they do it to help plan the nursery, anticipate a bris (Jewish ceremonial circumcision), pick a name (see Tip #66), have a sense of control, or plan for medical reasons. It's a personal decision that only a couple can make. I think we chose not to find out because my older brother didn't find out—anticipating, speculating, and coming up with names for both sexes was entertaining.

Just know that if you want to wait, it's not as big a hassle as some people lead you to believe. If you do wait, some people might pressure you and want to know. It might be family, it might be friends, it might be your pregnant partner—you should stick to what you believe. If a relative pressures you (like a parent), that person needs to back off. Unless there's a compelling reason—like someone is ill, someone is leaving for a military tour, or some other extreme circumstance—this isn't anyone's decision but yours. Give the people around you permission to be upset if you refuse to find out the sex. There are some things in the world that are no one else's business and this is one of those things. You and your partner get to decide.

Now, if you want to know and she doesn't want to know, or she wants to know and you don't want to know, you have a real problem. Some couples will have one partner find out and not tell the other. Some couples will find out and not tell family or friends (family and friends can get annoyed if you keep them guessing).

Some couples will not find

> I would have had them all be a surprise if I could go back…It was so much more emotional and exciting, especially with planned C-sections for the second and third child.
>
> —Jamie, sons, six and two, daughter, four

out but will have the caregiver notify retailers—*Be careful about this!* The last thing you want is to listen to a voice message from a sixteen-year-old part-time clerk explaining that *his* clothes will be ready for you to pick up when you leave the hospital. If you do confide in a vendor, make sure the information is kept secret. Make a deal and put it in writing—if the secret gets out, you get everything for free. (That should soften the blow.)

THE BOTTOM LINE:
What do you think? Boy? Girl? Wait and don't find out.

Tip #66
THE NAME GAME: What to Call Him or Her...

THE TIP:
If you have strong feelings about the name, make suggestions too. Don't just have her come up with names and shoot them all down.

THE STORY:
My husband and I argued a lot over the name. I didn't expect him to care, but he cared very much. I wanted him to make a list of names he liked, and I'd do the same. He preferred to have me make a list and then he would shoot down names I liked. That was a disaster because he shot down every name until about a week before each of our daughters was born.

> We eliminated any name that either one of us could bash.
> —*Cathy, sons, four months and three and a half*

This is one area where both partners should have equal say. I know one couple where the husband hates the son's name. The boy is now five and the father still talks about how he hates the name.

—*Tracy, son, three, daughter, twelve months*

It's the reason we found out the sex early so we could only argue over one set of names. We found a way to be much more efficient at arguing.

—*Carey, daughters, two and twenty-four months*

✳✳✳

It's one of the biggest decisions a parent can make. What to call the baby?

The name you choose will impact your child's entire life. There are no current laws preventing you from picking any name you choose. You can name a child a direction (North), a fruit (Apple), or Harlan (that's me). A bad name could turn your baby to a life of crime, isolation, and resentment. A good name can lead a child down the path of prosperity, happiness, and endless joy. It's really that big (but not really).

As the expectant father of a first child, you will find that your vote might not have as much power. In the words of one new mom, "For us, my vote was worth two, and his worth one. A veto from me and the name is gone." It's safe to assume that your pregnant partner will likely have the last word. And that word will be the baby's name.

It's hard to argue with

It's like choosing a restaurant. Give your wife three or four choices that you like and let her pick the winner. Make sure to reject anything you hate right away. Don't waiver.

—*AJ, son, eighteen months*

this thinking. (You can try to, but it's never a good idea to argue with a pregnant woman.) If your partner took your last name when you got married, the idea that you also get to pick the first name when it already gets your last name makes it a tough sell. You can argue that if the baby is a girl, her last name will be history when she gets married. So the first name is the only lasting name. While this might be true, you're not the one gaining the weight, tolerating raging hormones, puking, and pushing out a kid from between your legs. If you're lucky, you can get a middle name and naming rights to the second born. If we lived in the 1800s there wouldn't be a question; you would get naming rights to everything. But we live in the 2000s and men are equal partners (or just one notch slightly below equal). (**Note:** This is NOT true in all cases. Some women are cool with whatever name you will choose.)

TOP BABY BOY NAMES IN 2012:

1. Jacob
2. Mason
3. Ethan
4. Noah
5. William
6. Liam
7. Jayden
8. Michael
9. Alexander
10. Aiden

TOP BABY GIRL NAMES IN 2012:

1. Sophia
2. Emma
3. Isabella
4. Olivia
5. Ava
6. Emily
7. Abigail
8. Mia
9. Madison
10. Elizabeth

THINGS TO CONSIDER WHEN PICKING A NAME:

- Will the name result in teasing? Visit a class of eighth graders and ask them to make up hurtful nicknames for the name. You can also pick up the book *The Baby Name Wizard: A Magical Method for Finding the Perfect Name for Your Baby* (by Laura Wattenberg). In addition to some cool naming strategies, there is a ranking of how easy it is for a kid to be teased with each particular name.

> I don't want to hear about my friend's brother's girlfriend's aunt who has the same name and is a complete failure as a human being.
>
> —*Jessica, daughter, three, thirty-six weeks pregnant*

- How common is the name? Visit the social security website and check out the list of names dating back to 1879 (www.ssa.gov/OACT/babynames/).

Harlan was the 824th most popular name in 1973 (when I was born). In addition, check out www.NameBerry.com—you'll never look at choosing a name the same way again.

- Who do we name the kid after? Some couples of mixed faiths might find their cultures clash when it comes to naming. Some people will use the first letter or name of a deceased relative, some will use the first letter or name of a living relative, some will use the whole name, some the name of a parent, some will go with junior, II, or III (although it helps if there is a II before having a III).

- How do we spell it? Consider the name Amy. You can spell it the traditional way, *Amy*, or you can spell it a fancy way: *Aymhee, Aeayme, Aimknee* (silent *kn*), *Aymeeee, Aemhee,* or *Aaamhee.* While all these other spellings prove that you're incredibly clever (maybe not), they can also make life incredibly complicated for your kid. Yes, an interesting name with a spelling that needs to be repeated several times can make for a great conversation piece, but there are other things to talk about. If you do choose an alternative spelling, just make sure you know how to spell it.

TESTING THE NAMES

Naming your child is a personal decision. But still, there will be a time during the name search when you might want other people's feedback. Usually, these people are friends and family. Be cautious when vetting names. You'll discover that most people have some association with a name that you love. Your first choice might be the name of an ex-boyfriend who cheated, a sadistic boss who fired someone, a friend doing time, or the name of someone's pet golden retriever or cockatoo. If you love the name, it doesn't matter if anyone else loves it (other than your partner). The name will grow on the people around you. Once the baby is born, the name takes on an entirely different meaning.

If you want feedback, a safe way is to ask the people closest to you to share names starting with the letter you're considering using for a name. For example, if you're using the letter *H*, ask if anyone has any *H* names they love or don't love. Listen closely and keep your names a secret. Once you gauge the feedback, you can

NAMING RIGHTS (THE DAY MAY COME)

Depending on how early you are in the pregnancy, there may be an opportunity to fund your child's future by selling his or her naming rights. Let's say Cheetos wanted to promote their Cheetos Flamin' Hot Crunchy Snack brand. This would make my son's legal name "Cheetos Flamin' Hot Crunchy Cohen." This could be worth millions of dollars in exposure for Cheetos over my son's lifetime. And if Cheetos Flamin' Hot Crunchy Cohen were to run for student council, become a star athlete, or end up on TV, radio, or in print… we're talking huge dollars.

make your decision privately and tell no one until the birth. Let the world be surprised when they hear it.

PRENATAL NAMES

There are some people who will name their baby and refer to the baby by name before he or she is born. I'm not one of them. If you aren't either, here's a piece of advice: we created a prenatal name for our babies. I'm a big fan of it. You can create ridiculous names that take on personal meaning. Our daughter's prenatal name was "Harlephanie," a combination between Harlan and Stephanie (like "Brangelina"). Our second baby's name was "Happy HaHa." Our third baby's name was #3. (Yes, wildly creative, I know.)

THE BOTTOM LINE:
Hagina is not a good name.

Tip #67
HANGING OUT WITH HER BELLY: Talking, Singing, Touching, Petting, Patting, Painting, and Listening to It

THE TIP:
Take pictures—lots of pictures.

THE STORY:
One of the funniest moments of the pregnancy had to be when I was at about twenty-eight weeks along. My hubby would not stop staring at my tummy. Even though he sees me every day, he claims my tummy became ginormous

> When he rubs my belly, it reassures me that he likes me. I know he loves me. It is the fact that he is touching *me* that makes me feel happy.
>
> —*Nancy, fifteen weeks pregnant*

overnight. He then grabbed the camera and took pictures of it from every angle…I thought it was hilarious because he was behaving as if he just found out I was pregnant. I didn't mind that he used the word *ginormous* because he was so cute about it. He was 100 percent fascinated. I guess it really sunk in at that moment.

—*Amanda, daughters, six months and three*

***

> I currently sing to the baby twice a week. I put on a ten- to fifteen-minute concert. My best song is "Nose, Nose, Jolly Red Nose."
>
> —*Jeff, twenty-six weeks pregnant*

If you think she's big now, wait until she's about to give birth. It will look as if she consumed a small animal. It's huge. Whatever you do, don't tell her how huge *it* is and poke *it* with your finger. The *it* is attached to her, and she will associate these words with how she looks. When in awe, say things like, "You're so pregnant and so beautiful." Always throw in the qualifier after the amazement part.

By the time she arrives in the third trimester, you should be able to feel the baby kick. You'll get a little push, a finger, a toe, a knee, a foot, a hand, and a head. In the early stages, she'll feel it before you do. She'll want you to feel it, but you won't be able to feel it. She'll put your hand

LISTENING TO HER BELLY

You can feel it, you can talk to it, and you can just listen to it. We used a listening device that she placed just under the navel. There were two pairs of headphones (one for me and one for her). From the moment the monitor is activated, you're supposed to hear the magic of your baby's heartbeat in the womb. Beware of these listening devices. While it's supposed to be a magical experience, it can be anxiety-provoking if you do listen too early in the pregnancy or position the microphone in the wrong place on her belly.

That Magic Marker Line on Her Belly: You might notice a dark line appear from her belly button to her pubic area. It's called the linea nigra, and it's a result of the hormonal changes and increased pigment. Some women's are darker than others. This too will slowly disappear over time once the baby is born.

Her Massive Belly Button: As the uterus expands and puts pressure on the navel, her belly button will protrude. Once the baby is born, the navel will return to form.

on her belly and say, "Feel that? Feel it?" And you'll be like, "No."

After about forty-five minutes of trying and spasms in

DOCUMENTING HER BIG BELLY

Every few weeks or so, take a picture of her belly. Have her stand in the same place and in the same pose and outfit. At the end of the pregnancy, frame some of the photos and give them to her as a gift (a very reasonable push present). You can also have professional pictures taken at a studio of her and her naked belly (it's probably better if you kept yours covered).

your arm from holding it steady, you'll give up trying to feel it. This will go on for weeks. She'll call you over and over again, and all you'll feel is her big belly. Eventually, after weeks of trying, you'll feel something, and it will be the coolest thing ever. Once you feel the baby moving, you'll know she isn't making this whole thing up for attention. She's really pregnant.

At around weeks twenty-seven to twenty-eight, the baby's hearing will be completely developed. This means you can talk to it, sing to it, and do things with it. Keep in mind that you need to talk like the baby has a hearing problem in order to get through the swishing, popping, and whooshing of your partner's stopped-up gassy intestines.

Research has proven that

> I was surprised by just how large her stomach actually got. Hard to believe someone so small can get a belly that big.
> —Brad, son, twenty-four months, twenty-two weeks pregnant

babies can identify voices in utero. Speaking to the belly can be a great way to introduce yourself and begin a relationship. Consider playing music, reading books, or just making up stories while

chatting with the baby in her belly. Remember, though, that while the baby belongs to you too, her belly is still hers. She might not be into a live concert or storytelling session, so check in and reserve a time to hang out with her belly.

THE BOTTOM LINE:

When you're done having fun and playing with her belly, invite her to have fun and play with yours. It's only polite.

Tip #68
HANGING OUT WITH THE GUYS: Respecting Your Designated Pregnant Driver's Hours

THE TIP:

When she tells you to go out, make sure she really means it.

THE STORY:

My wife and I had a very active social life before she got pregnant. While she was pregnant, she couldn't go out like she used to. One night in particular, she told me to go out and have a good time. She hung out with the wife of the guy I went out with. I came back around 3:00 a.m., and she was waiting for me—upset. She couldn't understand how I could stay out so late. She then told me that she really didn't want me to go out, but she didn't realize this when she told me to go out. She was tired and irritated because I left her to entertain someone all night (although they were sleeping when we got back). I explained that I would have stayed home, but I couldn't know what she wanted because she didn't tell me what she wanted. Her problem was that I should have chosen to be at home, and if I went out, I should have known to come home earlier. From that point forward, I asked her to tell me what she wanted and not to be mad if she changes her mind after she tells me what she wants. She agreed.

—Jon, daughter, four months

✳✳✳

Having a social life is like placing a beer bottle on your partner's pregnant belly (not recommended)—it takes balance. It's balancing her need to know that you love her and your need to have a life independent of her.

Going out without her isn't like it was before she was pregnant. How late you stay out, how much you can drink, and what you can and can't do when you come home will not be the same. The more you can spoil her and pay attention to her, the easier it will be for her to encourage you to go out with the guys.

> Don't come home drunk out of your mind. It's really annoying and it reminds a woman that her life has drastically changed, but his hasn't.
>
> *—Ashley, daughter, twelve months*

PLAN A DADCHELOR PARTY

A new ritual for first-time fathers similar to a bachelor party, but with pregnant strippers (just kidding about the pregnant strippers). This rite of passage gives guys a chance to get together to share tips, drink beer from baby bottles, and indulge their selfish desires before becoming a role model. Read more: www.huffingtonpost.com/2011/06/13/dadelor-parties-celebrate-first-time-fathers_n_875968.html

Again, it's all about balance. And balance can mean:

- Taking her out on dates more than you go out with the guys on your own. It also means that when you are out with her on a date, ask if she minds before you order a drink (she can't). This is a classy move—unless you get to the point where you've had so much to drink that you can't put the words together to ask her for another or vomit. Then the balance has shifted the wrong way.
- That when she offers to be your designated driver, you don't call her at 2:00 a.m. to pick you up. A tired and nauseous pregnant woman doesn't want to pick up you and your drunk, smoky, stinking friends from a club with hot women who look like they're trying to get pregnant. The chances of her thinking

> Respect that she may want to go home earlier than you do.
> —*Carey, daughters, one month and two*

AND NOW, ANOTHER ACCIDENTAL ASSHOLE MOMENT

My husband asked me if he could go to Vegas two weeks before I was due. I asked him, "Are you serious?" He said, "Yes." I thought it was a joke. I told him to do whatever he wanted assuming he would never want to go. Well, then his friends bought him a ticket. He said he was going. I was shocked and horrified. Thankfully, at the last second, he realized Vegas two weeks before the due date wasn't worth the gamble.

—Blanca, son, six, daughter, four

this is funny are about as good as the chances of you getting lucky when you get home.

- That when she encourages you to go out with the guys, make a small gesture before you leave her alone. Small things like making her dinner, getting a movie, or recording her favorite shows mean you care.
- Not taking advantage of her. If she allows you to have drinks at the baby shower, don't get wasted. If she lets you go to the baseball game in her third trimester, come home after the game (not the next morning). If she lets you have friends over to play cards, don't smoke cigars and keep her up.
- That if you're planning to

My wife encouraged me to party, as she was happy to be my designated driver during all three of her pregnancies.

—Matt, daughter, ten, sons, seven and three

fly to Vegas for a bachelor party when she's in her 39th week, make it a one-way ticket, because she won't be there when you get back from your trip. There's just no way that's cool, man…

THE BOTTOM LINE:

Don't get so drunk you accidentally fall asleep and miss the birth. Bad. Very bad.

Tip #69
ULTRASOUND FOR KICKS: A Home Movie of Baby Hanging Out in the Womb

THE TIP:

I'm not sure we would have done it to determine the sex, but after having gone through the experience, I think an additional ultrasound at a center is a special experience for anyone—especially with your first baby.

THE STORY:

The hospital technician said, "I think I see a bulge, but can't say for sure." That wasn't good enough for us! The baby wasn't cooperating and getting into a good position to determine the sex. So we scheduled an appointment at a specialty ultrasound center (not in a mall). I did not ask if they were certified technicians, but I think it was explained in the literature they provided that this was not a medical facility. We chose the package that gave us a twenty-minute session, four printed photos, a DVD (set to music, which ended up being pretty cool), and gender determination.

This cost around $100, maybe a little more (they have several packages). When we got there, they took us into a comfortable room that had an ultrasound machine and a big projection screen (very cool—we were able to see images much better). It was just like having an ultrasound at the hospital, except once she found a good angle, she would switch it to the 3-D or 4-D image and we could see every feature. I thought it would be kind of creepy, but it was pretty cool. She confirmed the baby was a boy, explained what we were seeing (much more than the technician at the hospital did). She was *really* nice and excited for us, which made all the difference. The hospital technician was not very warm, which didn't help our experience. Having the DVD recording was great because we were able to show our parents and friends who were interested. The recording was set to lullaby music, very sweet. I would definitely recommend this.

—Heather, son, two months

＊＊＊

> All these people would tell me horror stories about birth, women screaming, bad things happening, and babies getting sick, but none of it ever happened to us.
>
> *—Kevin, daughter, two, twenty-eight weeks pregnant*

Just because your doctor is done giving ultrasounds doesn't mean you can't get some bonus footage. Stores like Fetal Fotos and Prenatal Peek offer parents elective ultrasounds. Expectant parents can get detailed photos and see live-motion color images of their unborn babies inside the womb. Some services can even broadcast on the Internet.

I got a taste of 3-D/4-D imaging (similar to what is used at these places) during one of our doctor's visits. What I saw was a bunch of questions. The skin looked bumpy and scary. Shadows looked like weird growths. I was completely unsure of what I was seeing. The only thing that made it comfortable to watch was the doctor telling me not to worry about it.

When it comes to elective ultrasounds, you'll find a wide range of opinions. The FDA issued the following caution against prenatal portraits: "Ultrasound is a form of energy, and even at low levels, laboratory studies have shown it can produce physical effects in tissue, such as jarring vibrations and a rise in temperature." Although there is no evidence that these physical effects can harm a fetus, the FDA says the fact that these effects exist means that prenatal ultrasounds can't be considered completely innocuous.

Another reason some advise against commercial ultrasounds is that some operators have discovered abnormalities or complications (read the article "Avoid Fetal 'Keepsake' Images, Heart Monitors" at www.fda.gov /downloads/ForConsumers /ConsumerUpdates/ucm 095602.pdf). There's also

> In a family with two dads, most everything you will encounter is mom-centric. I was not prepared for all the unsolicited advice from total strangers. It can be annoying if not intrusive. A friend offered the best advice. He told me, "This is your child and you know him better than anyone else. Let that advice go in one ear and right out the other."
>
> —Oren, son, seven

the risk of seeing something that you think looks like a problem but isn't a problem.

If you want snapshots, consult your care provider and consider doing it immediately following an appointment with your doctor. You can also inquire about recording the ultrasound during your doctor's visits. If you do opt for the bonus ultrasound, just let your caregiver tell you that everything is *perfect* first, so shadows don't make you crazy.

THE BOTTOM LINE:

The only thing better than home movies are home movies from inside the womb. Perfect for the kid's wedding video (you can show it at the rehearsal dinner).

Tip #70
UNSOLICITED ADVICE: The Things Some People Will Share with You

THE TIP:

If someone offers you advice and hands you a videotape to go along with it, thank them, and hand it back. Tell them to keep any graphic home videos with their own personal collection.

THE STORY:

When we got pregnant with our first, my sister-in-law ran downstairs to get a video for us. It was labeled "family," which I thought was interesting. She said, "This is a video-tape of me giving birth. When you feel comfortable, watch it. It should help answer your questions." We were about five months along when we popped the tape in. The first shot was of my sister-in-law and her husband sitting at a table—she wasn't pregnant or anything. We thought it was the wrong tape…Then there was a flash of static and the screen cut to the moment of truth. The entire screen was 100 percent vagina and the baby's head coming out of it. When I say 100 percent, I mean the *entire* screen was vagina. It was vagina and orb. I felt like I was watching an IMAX movie. I had never seen crowning at that point and my first question to my wife was, "What the F**K is that?" She explained. What I admired was the videography. My brother-in-law stayed with the shot all the way through the pushing. When the baby was coming out, I felt like I was there for the actual birth. The camera cut away just in time to show a rush of fluid gush out, which was more than I could take. My wife was crying because it was such a beautiful moment; I was somewhere between horrified and titillated. When our baby was born, I stayed up by my wife's shoulders and didn't videotape it. I had seen enough.

—*Corey, daughters, two and four*

***

Friends, family, strangers, medical professionals, priests, rabbis, coworkers, bus drivers, and people in stores, elevators, airplanes, and restaurants will all offer you unsolicited advice. Some advice will be helpful, some absurd, some offensive, some shocking, and some funny. When

> Have her show you what you should bring, not what you think you should bring.
> —*Scott, daughter, ten months*

people give you annoying, wrong, and stupid tips (see Tip #16 for a refresher), just nod your head and say thank you. Then tweet it and share it on Facebook (as long as they aren't your Facebook friends or followers on Twitter). And now, common clichés and advice friends, family, and strangers will share with you again and again.

"LIFE IS GOING TO CHANGE…"

Yes, no shit, Zen Buddhist Master. It's not that people say, "Life will change." It's *how* they say it. They make it seem so ominous and foreboding. And then when you say, "Yeah, I know it's going to change," they say it again, "No, you don't understand, it's *really*

IT'S OKAY TO QUESTION CONVENTION

I read a *New York Times* article about infant potty training which explained how in many parts of the world, potty training starts at birth. I read the book *Infant Potty Training* and decided to try it at six weeks. People thought we were crazy. Even my husband resisted at first. That was until our seven-week-old pooped and peed in the potty. Everyone was shocked that it could work. Then, all of a sudden, I wasn't so crazy.
—Stephanie, daughter, twenty months, eight weeks pregnant

going to change!" And you're like, "Right, I heard you, it's going to change." Then they get all excited, "*No, man, you don't hear me. It's* really *going to change.*" (Then you will want to smack them.) I'll tell the truth. It will change, but it can change for the better. I'll touch more on this in Tip #92 (just after the baby is born). For advice on how to handle the "It's Going to Change Advice Guy," check out The Bottom Line. But don't let anyone freak you out about the change. It takes time to adjust, but once you're there, it's the *very best change*.

"THIS ISN'T HOW WE DID IT…"

You might be doing something differently than your friends, family, or parents. And doing something differently means opening yourself up to criticism. If there's solid research and it's safe, why not try something different? Doing things differently than the way they've always been done doesn't mean doing something wrong—it means there could be another, better way to do something. Don't be surprised when people question you. When they do, don't try to convince them that you've chosen a better path. Trust that they'll see what you see and then say, "I can't believe it, but you were right…" And even if they don't say you're right, you're making your own choices, and that's what it means to be a parent.

"I HEARD THE MOST HORRIBLE STORY…"

People are going to come up to you or partner and tell you stories that you don't want to hear. These people deserve your compassion—they are complete morons. I'm not going to be one of these people, because really, there's no reason for you to be panicked. The majority of people will *not* experience a problem. Even if you do have some kind of problem, there will usually be answers. If you're expecting and someone starts talking to you about a tragedy or complication, tell them you'd rather not hear about it. Most of the time, they have no idea what they're doing and will stop once they realize their mistake.

THE BOTTOM LINE:

If someone tells you that life is going to change one more time, respond with, "What do you mean?" Keep saying, "What do you mean?" after each explanation until the guy offering advice passes out from exhaustion trying to explain this to you or jumps out the window in frustration because you don't get it.

Tip #71
PACKING FOR THE TRIP: Everything You Need to Bring for the Both of You

THE TIP:
Make her a music mix and take it with you.

THE STORY:

> Do *not* overpack. We brought so much extra stuff that we didn't need. You will end up shuttling everything from room to room when you really should be focusing on your wife's comfort.
> —*Eric, daughter, twenty months*

A friend of ours told us that it was helpful to have music in the delivery room. They brought their iPod with them. When we went on the hospital tour, they also told us it would be a good idea to bring music. One night, right around week thirty-five, we put together a playlist for

KEEP THE GAS TANK
FULL (or not less than
half). Make sure your car
never gets near empty
during the third trimester.
Pulling off to get gas on
the way to the hospital
will turn you into an
accidental asshole.

the labor. It was just a nice night together. We picked out some of his favorites and some of mine. The hospital had a player in the room so we didn't need to bring one with us. The music helped me relax. Now, whenever I hear "Good People" by Jack Johnson, my eyes tear up.

—*Mandy, daughter,
two months*

***

Unless you're having this baby in your bedroom, you're going to need to pack a bag.

Pack early and pick a comfortable clean outfit for the big day. I know thinking about your wardrobe might sound ridiculous, but you'll want to be comfortable. And you'll see yourself in the clothes you pack for the rest of your life. If you're a last-minute packer, make sure you have a list together and clean clothes set aside.

For example, if you wear hats, make sure you wash the one you take with you. If you live by the rule that denim isn't dirty until it smells, you might want to change your rule. These are the clothes you'll be wearing when you hold your clean, pristine, pure baby for the first time. The baby will be resting on your chest, lying on your lap, and drooling on your clothes. You'll want them to be clean.

Considering that some hospitals were designed before

dads were so involved in the process, your needs are not always factored into the floor plan. You might find out that you have nowhere to sleep. Ask the hospital or birthing facility where new dads sleep. You may have to bring an air mattress or your own pillow.

On the next page, I've included a list of things to pack. Also, check with someone you know who has given birth at the same place. Ask the question, "What do you wish you brought that you needed?" If you don't know someone, you can stop by the facility and ask some dads hanging out there. If you can avoid packing too much stuff, you'll be thrilled when you see all the other stuff you'll accumulate during your visit. If you forget something, you, a friend, or a family member can always run out to get it. The most important items are the birth plan, her stuff, and your pregnant partner. Make sure you bring her or you'll have a big problem.

The following are suggestions from new moms and dads. Following these suggestions, I've provided a list of things I think you should bring. If you're in a hurry, you can rip out the page and use it as a checklist when frantically packing.

Things to keep in mind for her:

- Don't take everything on the list from class. I never touched half of it!
- Take some comfy clothes and a baseball hat if you're a hat person.
- Don't forget her makeup, if she wears it.
- Avoid smelly lotions or perfumes (not good if she's trying to breastfeed).
- Pack light—she will feel too gross and dirty to wear the cute new pajamas that you bought.

- Bring her own pillow.
- Pack some books or magazines for her to read.
- Take footies, slippers, or warm socks; consider flip-flops for the shower.
- Pack her favorite snacks.
- Bring a bottle of water (you never know).
- Bring ear plugs! (This is the best advice I have ever received.)

For baby:

- Install the car seat (don't forget the car seat!!!).
- Pack a baby outfit for pictures.
- Pack one special outfit for the trip home.

THE BOTTOM LINE:
Bring your pregnant partner.

Tip #72
PATERNITY LEAVE: A Paid (or Unpaid) Vacation with Your New Family

THE TIP:
Take at least a week off. If you can take another consecutive week and still get paid, take it.

THE STORY:
When the baby was born, I took a week off. And then within the month, I took another week. It was our first baby, and it was a little rough—she needed the help. We

CUT HERE

HARLAN'S PACKING LIST

_ Directions
_ The birth plan
_ Hospital paperwork/medical records
_ Car seat
_ Pediatrician's information
_ The Happiest Baby on the Block book and/or DVD
_ iPod, iPad, music player, and speaker (if the hospital has a player)
_ Snack foods (trail mix, bars, nuts, and her favorites)
_ Toiletries for two nights
_ Bathing suit (in case you help her in the shower and the nurse comes in)
_ Change of clothes for three days and two nights (make sure the clothes are clean)
_ Comfortable shoes (you'll do a lot of standing)
_ A clean hat (if you're a hat person; don't forget to wash it)
_ Email addresses of people to whom you want to send birth updates
_ Laptop computer and power cord
_ Digital camera or video camera, charger, extra memory card, extra tapes
_ Cell phone and cell phone charger
_ Roll of quarters for vending machines
_ Her suitcase and reading materials
_ An extra bag to haul stuff home
_ Disinfectant wipes
_ If packing for her—comfortable clothes, not nice underwear, slippers, toiletries, contact solution (if she wears contacts), glasses, and an outfit to go home in
_ This page of the book (or the whole book)

get two weeks, but not necessarily two consecutive weeks. In an ideal world, if you could take two consecutive weeks, that's great. I don't think many people can take off for two weeks. But I think the first week is necessary. During the second week, there isn't a lot you can do, unless she's struggling with her health or the baby isn't cooperating. A week is enough. Fortunately both of our kids were easy babies. The second week, I just hung out. I played golf once. When the kid was sleeping, I would help around the house, but after you have the second one, the routine is so much easier. By the end of the week, I was ready to get back to my normal life.

—Kevin, daughter, eleven months, son, three

✳✳✳

Plan to take more time than you'll need.

If you're not a full-time dad, you'll need to figure out how long you'll stay at home once the baby is born. There's paid leave (vacation days, paternity leave, sick days) and unpaid leave. How much time you take is a personal decision. Not everyone has the luxury of taking time off. But if you do have the option, take advantage of all your time.

Having a baby can be physically and emotionally exhausting. Taking care of the baby takes time to get comfortable. Depending on

> Today was my first day back after the longest stretch I'd been away from work. Throughout the day, my wife emailed me pictures of what they were doing. It was just awesome. It helped ease my transition. It was nice to feel like I was still involved.
>
> *—Chris, son, two weeks*

your health insurance provider and the delivery, your partner may be back home in less than forty-eight hours. If she has a C-section, she'll be in the hospital longer, and her recovery will be longer and harder. Regardless of the ease of the delivery, when she gets home, you need to be a co-parent. This means that you'll play an equal role as long as you're both home. She might not be able to walk up stairs, pick up the baby, or do some of the basic things. So if you don't have the luxury of taking time off, make sure she has a family member or close friend who can be there during the first weeks.

SURPRISE, IT COULD BE A C-SECTION

Take more time than you will need. Considering one-third of women have C-sections, you might need to do more than you expected. C-sections require more time. You can always go back to work early.

Even if everything goes spectacularly smoothly, you're still going to be exhausted the first week, maybe too exhausted to work. If the baby is sleeping in your room, it might wake up crying to feed every couple of hours. If you were to go back to work, getting up for work wouldn't involve getting up because you'd never get to sleep. Regardless of who is the primary caregiver, it can take a good week to develop a routine and get comfortable with the baby. Until you've worked out the routine, leaving her alone or her leaving you alone can be too much. Besides, during the first week, someone needs to be around to run out for diaper cream, a different kind of bottle, dinner, and groceries. She will need you.

Another reason to take time off is that there is always

a chance that something won't go as smoothly as you had hoped. In case that happens, make sure you can be there. If you can set aside two weeks, that's even better. You might find out that your benefits include a week or two or three of paid leave—maybe even longer. For example, both new mothers and fathers at Yahoo! can now take eight weeks of paid parental leave, and the mothers can take an additional eight weeks. What's more, new parents will also receive $500 to buy items like groceries and clothes. It's part of a slate of new benefits "to support the happiness and well-being of Yahoos and their families," the company confirmed via email.

If your place of employment doesn't have paid leave for men and does have paid leave for women, there's nothing wrong with making some noise. Corporate culture is beginning to recognize the role of men, but it's still a slow go. Check out a video by a friend of mine who decided to take matters in his own hands: www.DadsExpectingToo.com.

If you don't have benefits that will pay you for paternity leave, you might qualify for unpaid leave. Under the Family and Medical Leave Act (FMLA), if you work at a large office (fifty or more employees within a 75-mile radius) and you've worked for your employer for at least twelve months and for at least 1,250 hours during the previous year (which comes out to twenty-five hours per week for fifty weeks), you might be protected under the law. There are some exceptions, but you can check it out by visiting the U.S. Department of Labor's website: www.dol.gov.

The best advice is to check with your human resources department and review your benefits.

THE BOTTOM LINE:

This time together is priceless. Take as much as you can afford.

11

LABOR AND DELIVERY PREP TIME

Things to Help Prepare You for Labor and Delivery

Tip #73
THE BIRTH PLAN: How It Will All Go Down...

THE TIP:
I wish we had planned better for our first.

THE STORY:
When I was in labor, I was unable to speak for myself. I was so self-absorbed (in the labor process) that I couldn't think about much else, let alone articulate my thoughts to the medical personnel. I wish I had known during my first labor how things would go so we could have prepared better. We would have reviewed exactly what my preferences

were and how he would address certain issues with the nurses and doctors. The second time around, we went over exactly what we wanted, and it was a far more comfortable experience and so much better.

—*Lesha, sons, seven months and three and a half*

***

The average man's birth plan:

- Go to the hospital.
- Count contractions.
- Cut the cord.
- Take pictures.
- Post them online.
- Celebrate.

As a first-time dad, it's hard to plan when you don't know what you need to know.

For our first child, we didn't have a birth plan. For our second, we had a plan (but didn't write it down). For our third, we plan to use the previous plan with some modifications. That's because once we went through this process the first time, we learned that we have a lot more control over the birth than we realized. We set the tone and make the rules. We can decide what medication we want (or don't want). We can decide how quickly we want things to progress. We can choose what happens after the baby is born. It might be routine for the caregivers, but not for us.

Had something unexpected happened or had my wife

been unable to answer questions, it would have been my call to execute the birth plan. If she were unavailable to answer questions about the delivery, I would be left to use my best judgment—and using my own judgment during delivery is a frightening prospect. That's why it's helpful to have a birth plan in place before her water breaks.

When you write a birth plan and discuss it in advance, you can refer to it during the delivery. And if something surprising pops up, you can have some direction. Look at the birth plan as if you're the head coach preparing for game day. In order to plan, you need to know the fundamentals of the game. Becoming knowledgeable and having a plan can relieve some of the stress that comes with facing the unknown during this experience.

Make sure you talk about this plan early in the third trimester. Imagine how it will play out. And now some topics to discuss with your pregnant partner and caregiver before entering the birthing arena:

2011 BIRTH FACTS AND STATS

- Number of births: 3,953,590
- Fertility rate: 63.2 births per 1,000 women aged 15-44 years
- Percent born low birth weight: 8.1%
- Cesarean delivery rate: 32.8 %
- Percent born preterm: 11.73%
- Percent unmarried: 40.7%

(Source: www.cdc.gov /nchs/data/nvsr/nvsr62 /nvsr62_01.pdf)

- Where you will be having this baby (hospital, birthing center, home)?
- When should you go to the birthing location?
- If your doctor isn't available, who will be the doctor doing the delivery?
- Do you have any preferences regarding the birthing environment (music, lighting, etc.)?
- What kind of snacks and other things should you bring?
- Who will be allowed in the delivery room?
- What are the facility's postpartum visiting hours and rules?
- Does she want pain medication? If so, what kind and when?
- Does she want Pitocin? (This helps get the contractions going.)
- Does she want a mirror to assist in pushing? (This helps some women stay motivated.)
- Where does she want you to stand?
- Under which circumstances is an episiotomy performed? (An episiotomy is a procedure in which the area between the birth canal and the anus is cut.)
- Does she want to be mobile or in bed? Preferred position for pushing?
- Does she want a birthing ball? Back massage should back labor start?
- What will your role be in the labor and delivery?
- Do you want to cut the umbilical cord?
- Do you want the baby to have skin-on-skin contact immediately following delivery?
- If having a C-section, what is the procedure? Are you allowed in the room?

- If having a C-section, will she hold the baby immediately following delivery?
- Once the baby is born, what's the procedure? Do you have any preferences?
- Will she breastfeed or formula feed?
- Does the facility have a lactation consultant?
- What are you doing with the cord blood?
- Will the baby sleep in the room with you or in the nursery?
- Have you already chosen a pediatrician?
- Do you have email addresses and phone numbers so you can spread the news?
- Who will be point person on the outside to share news and info?
- Do you have a car seat in the car ready to take the baby home?

THE BOTTOM LINE:

If you're reading this on the way to the hospital, tear out this page and write some of the answers down. Or you can ask your partner these questions in between contractions during early labor.

Tip #74
THE BIRTH CLASS: The Final Exam Will Be Here before You Know It

THE TIP:

When attending your first relaxation class, make sure you are helping your wife to relax, not focusing on yourself.

THE STORY:

When we attended our first Lamaze-type class, the instructor went through a demo on how to give a massage. After going through the specifics, he told us that one of us should massage the other one. I had my wife go to work on my shoulders. It had been a long day, and I was feeling sore. We looked around the class and every other husband was rubbing his pregnant wife's shoulders. I was the only selfish asshole in the room getting a rubdown. We quickly switched positions.

—*Matt, daughter, ten, sons, seven and three*

✳✳✳

Welcome back to the classroom.

The birth class is a rite of passage that every expectant father should be required to experience at least once. There's no good reason *not* to go. Even the longest, most boring, and poorly instructed class has value. Some classes can be interesting, fast-paced, and entertaining. If you're assisting in a natural birth (no

We went to several classes, including infant CPR, Lamaze, and breastfeeding. All were interesting but could have been cut down by about a third as many hours.
—*Mike, son, three months*

pain medication and mini-
mal intervention), you'll
need to be more familiar
with and more involved
during all stages of labor.
Attending a birthing class
will be essential. Regardless
of your partner's birth plan,
the class will help you think
about what she will experience and how you can help.
The more familiar you are

CLASSROOM COURTESY

Turn off your cell phone
during class—no texting,
checking scores, or
doing anything other
than being in class
and with your partner,
unless she asks you to.

with what to expect, the easier it will be for you to remain
calm and offer support.

Since my wife planned on having a medicated delivery, my
role was more of support rather than coaching. We attended
two classes. One lasted about eight hours on a Saturday. The
other was an infant CPR class (*very* helpful, especially the
infant choking demo). During the all-day birth class, we
learned about the three stages of labor (more in Tip #84),
pain management, contractions (telling fake ones from real
ones), and some breathing and massaging techniques. We
were introduced to the fetal monitors. We talked as a group
about what excited us about the baby. We changed diapers.
We watched videos that were less graphic than I expected (I
was disappointed). We also participated in a grab bag that
included items that patients will encounter during the birth
process. I was fortunate enough to grab a super-absorbent
maxi pad used to soak up the blood and draining liquid
(lucky me). Someone else got pregnant woman underwear—
what she wears after delivery. (Not a turn-on.)

The most valuable part of the class for me was the hospital tour. Seeing the labor and delivery room, the fetal monitors, and the areas where the baby is examined and cleaned up gave me a clear picture of what to expect. Men are visual creatures—seeing things and being there helps us get a better feel for what's to come. If you can't make it to a class because of work or some other reason, at the very least get a tour of the labor and delivery rooms. Seeing where it will happen will give you a mental picture to help fill in some of the unknowns.

BONUS CLASS: TAKE INFANT CPR

My wife made me take an additional infant CPR class that included how to help a choking infant. She also required the grandparents and babysitter to attend. None of us wanted to go, but it was the *best* and most valuable thing. Take it. In the meantime, you can view an instructional video of infant CPR and a choking demonstration online at http://depts.washington.edu/learncpr/. For information on infant CPR classes, contact your local hospital or American Red Cross (www.redcross.org).

THE BOTTOM LINE:

Whether you go to class or not, the final exam is coming…

> Take a birthing/pregnancy class at a hospital. Even if you think you know what's going to happen, you'll still be surprised. You need to try to prepare for everything and anything. I was prepared for "the big show," but I was still shocked, amazed, and overwhelmed with emotion. I would say even if you are a tough guy, you might shed a tear.
>
> —*Brian, daughter, twelve months*

Tip #75
THE LABOR PARTNER: Helping Her Breathe, Push, and Relax

THE TIP:

It takes real engagement from the husband/partner to do it. The more I knew, the easier it was to be there for her.

THE STORY:

We followed the Bradley Method. My role was clear: to help my partner relax—that's at the heart of it. There's lots of prep time involved. We started taking classes in the fourth or fifth month. There's usually a series of twelve classes, but we did a four-course program. We practiced relaxation techniques at home. One exercise involved having her lie in bed and hold ice cubes in her hands. The idea was to practice relaxing her body while holding the ice. We probably did that five to ten times. We must have practiced other relaxation techniques at least twenty times. We would sink into the bed and find the least painful posture that strained the fewest muscles. She also practiced the birthing position on her side. Lying in certain positions that allow her to go deep into the contractions is part of it. What was most helpful to me was that being so involved helped me understand exactly what was going on during

> I remember them telling us in class that birth can be exhausting. We need to take breaks when she takes breaks. We need to sit down when we can. We need to eat and stay hydrated. We need to do all these things so when it matters, we'll be fresh.
>
> —Chris, son, twenty months

QUESTION: THE MOST HELPFUL THING HE DID FOR YOU DURING DELIVERY

ANSWERS:
- He coached, supported, put cool rags to my head, and massaged me.
- He brought me ice chips and encouraged me.
- He held my hand during transition labor, which is the worst.
- Nothing. The poor guy didn't know what to do.
- He stayed calm.
- He turned off the football game.
- He kept telling me that I was doing great.
- He stayed by my side the whole time.
- He was patient.
- He listened to what I needed.
- He timed the contractions.
- He massaged my back during back labor.
- He got the nurse and doctor when I asked.
- He made sure the birth plan was followed.
- He didn't argue with me.
- He told me I was strong.
- He was so amazing and attentive to me.
- He looked me in the eyes and kept me calm during my four hours of pushing.

the birth. I used to think childbirth was painful because a woman is pushing a giant thing through a small hole.

Really, it's the contractions that are painful. The Bradley Method explained how the muscles were working to open up the cervix. Labor wasn't just random pain. There was purpose. It's wonderfully empowering for us to have done this together and for me to be able to help her.

—*Peter, son, eighteen months*

✳✳✳

I panicked a couple weeks before delivery because I realized I had no idea what the hell I was supposed to do during labor. Never having been through it before, I didn't know how the sport of giving birth played out. And really, a coach who doesn't know the sport is not a good coach.

I can tell you that after doing this labor and delivery thing twice, we know what we like and don't like. The first time, we felt more like we were passengers on the birth train. We were tentative. And that's normal. The second time around, we offered directions and knew what we wanted. We did not want to be pressured. We knew my wife didn't want medicine to increase the pace of her contractions unless the baby's health was at stake. We knew we wanted time with the baby immediately after delivery. The first time, they whisked my daughter away, and I had to decide whether to stay with the baby or my wife. The second time, my son was placed right into my wife's arms following delivery. It was the best. The third time around, we decided if there are complications, we want the baby as close to my wife as possible during any treatment. Babies do their best close to mom, skin-to-skin.

When planning her labor and delivery, talk to friends

who have been there and done it. Ask them, "What are three things I need to know about labor?"

My answer: (1) Labor can be long for first-time parents. Pace yourself. It's a lot of hurry up and wait. (2) You are in charge. If you want answers and don't get them, press until you get them. No one cares as much as you. Sometimes things can get routine for the nurses and staff. (3) Always ask if something is unclear. Don't let anyone poke, prod, or test your partner (or the baby) without explaining the poke, prod, or test. Don't worry about being annoying. It's your job to know what is happening. You are an advocate for both your partner and your baby.

If your partner is having a natural birth, you'll have a bigger coaching role. And if you've gone through the twelve-week Bradley Method program, you'll be well prepared. You know how things should work. You'll have a birth plan in place. You know the plays. You will have practiced positions. You'll be ready for the main event.

Whether you call yourself a coach or a partner, it helps to know what's going on. This is where having a birth plan in place is helpful. Get an idea of what she wants and expects. Have a signal that will let you know you need to change what you're doing (like when she slaps you across the cheek). One woman will like to be massaged; another wants to be left alone. Some want music, others silence. Some will scream; others will push with quiet intensity.

> She just wanted to be left alone. My job for the first was to make sure there was a mirror there. My job for the second was to hold the camera, the camcorder, and her leg and to make sure the mirror was angled right for her.
>
> —Jim, daughter, two months, son, three

Some will want a cold towel; others will want nothing against their forehead. You'll figure it out.

Being a partner or coach means knowing what's happening and knowing what to expect. The more comfortable you can be with the uncomfortable part of labor, the easier it will be for you to remain calm and focused, which will ultimately help her stay calm and focused. I hope the rest of this book will help you become comfortable in the role you play.

THE BOTTOM LINE:

Attention coaches (and labor partners): doping *is* legal in this sport.

METHODS OF DELIVERY

The History of Lamaze

Lamaze is a philosophy of giving birth developed by Dr. Ferdinand Lamaze in 1951. The goal of Lamaze classes is to increase women's confidence in their ability to give birth. Lamaze classes teach women simple coping strategies for labor, including focused breathing. But Lamaze also teaches that breathing techniques are just one of the many things that help women in labor. Movement, positioning, labor support, massage, relaxation, hydrotherapy, and the use of heat and cold are some others. The Lamaze philosophy of birth is the centerpiece of Lamaze education, which teaches the following: (1) Birth is normal, natural, and healthy. (2) The experience of birth profoundly affects women and their families. (3) Women's inner wisdom guides them through birth. (4) Women's confidence and ability to give birth is either enhanced or diminished by the care provider and place of birth. (5) Women have the right to give birth free from routine medical interventions. (6) Birth can safely take place in homes, birth centers, and hospitals. (7) Childbirth education empowers women to make informed choices in health care, to assume responsibility for their health, and to trust their inner wisdom.

(Source: www.Lamaze.org)

The Bradley Method

In the late 1940s, Dr. Robert Bradley developed a method that embraced childbirth as a natural process that can be managed without pain medication and routine intervention. The Bradley Method is a twelve-week program that focuses on relaxation and pain management through natural means. Bradley believed that it takes months to prepare mentally, physically, and emotionally for childbirth. Bradley classes cover nutrition, exercise, approaches to improve comfort during pregnancy, the role of the coach, introductory information about labor and birth, advanced techniques for labor and birth, complications, C-sections, postpartum care, breastfeeding, and caring for the newborn baby.

Tip #76
WORKING THE DOOR: It's Like Being the Bouncer at Club Push

THE TIP:
Talk about who will be in the room ahead of time. Set boundaries early and avoid hurt feelings later.

THE STORY:
My wife and I talked about what would happen if things got difficult in the delivery room. She had gestational diabetes, so she was induced on her due date. The contractions were very slow at first, and her mom was in the room with us for the first six hours, just passing time. As things started to get intense, I started to feel uncomfortable. Her mom was sitting in the chair and not participating. I should mention that my wife wanted a natural delivery (with no medication), and her mom had expressed feelings of not understanding why anyone would want to experience pain. It was my decision to ask her to step out of the room. I told her that my wife would appreciate the privacy. She got a little defensive and wanted to ask my wife if she shared the same sentiment. My wife said the same thing, and her mom walked out in a huff. I walked into the waiting area and explained to her that I didn't mean to hurt her feelings. It wasn't a personal attack on her. There's a lot of emotion

> It never occurred to me that anyone else would be in the delivery room with us. My mother-in-law was disappointed when we informed her that she wouldn't be in there.
>
> —Irl, son, twenty-two months, twenty-eight weeks pregnant

and pain involved and I wanted to be respectful. She left the hospital and went home to clear her head. When she came back, my wife had gotten the epidural and things calmed down. We invited her mother back in the room for short periods of time, but she was much better when asked to leave now that we had established boundaries. It all worked out in the end.

—*Lawrence, daughter, seventeen months*

***

Not only are men in the delivery room, but we also control who gets in.

You're the guy who is in control of traffic during labor and delivery. Your partner will have the final say about who stays and goes, but she will be busy the day of the big event. Who gets access to the delivery room is her call (although, if she wants ex-boyfriends in attendance, that's crossing the line). You and your partner should discuss this when going over the birth plan (*before* she gives birth—it's not a conversation to have in the middle of labor).

If any of her choices make you uncomfortable or if you think the people affected by her choices will be uncomfortable, talk to them ahead of time. Set boundaries and make sure friends and family have reasonable expectations. If she doesn't want her mom in the room, she can talk to her mom ahead of time. If she

> She wanted to have a close friend in the delivery room with us. I didn't mind it. I was surprised how helpful it was to have someone else there.
>
> —*Kevin, daughter, two, thirty-six weeks pregnant*

doesn't want your parents in the room, you can talk to them about this. And just in case any family or friends who want to be in the room forget that they're not supposed to be in the room, put it in writing and include it in the birth plan in case you need to whip it

AVOID BIRTH ROOM BRAWLS

Have your partner tell the people closest to her who will be in the room with her LONG BEFORE her water breaks.

out. That birth plan can do all the talking for you. If you set the rules early, it shouldn't be a problem.

During my wife's labor, my parents and in-laws were allowed to hang out in the birthing room before the action. We told them ahead of time that we might ask them to leave at certain times. They were good listeners. When asked to come in, they came. When the labor started getting intense, we had to ask them all to leave, and they left. And yes, it can be uncomfortable telling your wife's parents to get out—not all parents like to be asked to leave when their daughter is in the midst of a medical procedure. That's why it helped to have already discussed this in advance.

The last thing you need is to battle a parent in the midst of delivery. If you have an older sibling who has gone through labor and delivery, family members might have similar expectations. Your pregnant partner might not do it the same way. Again, if you talk about this ahead of time, and everyone has the same expectations, you'll have one less thing to worry about the day of the delivery. Should plans change or someone get upset, or should someone start pushing his or her own agenda, bring them back to what this is about—your partner's comfort.

THE BOTTOM LINE:
No stun guns while working the door. Too tempting.

Tip #77
CORD BLOOD BANKING: Saving It Could Mean Saving a Life

THE TIP:
If you have a family history of a disease that is treatable with cord blood, look into cord blood banking.

THE STORY:
We decided to collect the cord blood for our second baby. I'm not sure why we didn't do it the first time—that's a question for my wife. I do know that we decided to do it because my wife has a family history of leukemia, and stem cells might be able to treat something like that. If banking had been around for my wife's relative, there might have been another option for treatment. We were never told about public banking or pressured into private banking. We made our decision based on having a family member with a disease.

> —Marc, son, fourteen months, daughter, four

> We chose to do public cord blood banking so that anyone could have access to the stem cells.
> —Amy, thirty-nine weeks pregnant

***

What are you going to do with the cord blood? Has anyone asked?

IMPORTANT: DO NOT THROW AWAY THAT CORD BLOOD
Visit www.marrow .org/Get_Involved /Donate_Cord_Blood /How_to_Donate/How _to_Donate.aspx.

If you're unfamiliar with cord blood, it's the stem cell-rich blood collected from the umbilical cord. Cord blood can potentially be used to treat leukemia, other cancers, blood disorders, and a number of other diseases. There are ongoing trials to test how cord blood can be used to treat other illnesses. Unlike adult stem cells, cord blood stem cells are biologically younger and more flexible. In twenty-seven states, cord blood education is now the law. In 2011, both Florida and Missouri passed state laws to educate expectant parents about cord blood banking. While most states require education, there is not always a requirement to discuss banking options. That's up to you.

You can do one of three things with the cord blood:

1. Nothing (a tragedy)
2. Store it in a private cord blood bank
3. Donate it to a public cord blood bank

1. DO NOTHING
We recycle plastic, paper, and garbage, but sadly, about 95 percent of people throw away their baby's cord blood. And it's because no one educates new parents on the potentially lifesaving advantages. This is slowly changing, but not fast

enough. You can bank either privately or publicly, or throw the cord blood away. But do not *throw your cord blood away*. If you're worried about costs, you can donate to a public bank for free. When it comes to private banking, call and explore payment plans and discounts.

2. STORE IT IN A PRIVATE CORD BLOOD BANK

When my daughter was born, we chose to do the private cord blood banking because it just seemed like another way to protect our unborn child. We did it again with my son's cord blood. We called up the 800 number and spoke to a salesperson. They sent us the collection kit and told us to bring it when we went to the hospital. We informed our doctor several weeks in advance of our decision. After our daughter was born, the doctor collected the blood and put it in the kit. I called the 800 number and a courier arrived at the hospital and sent it overnight to the storage facility. It was that easy.

While I have no regrets about our decision, I wish there had been more information and better guidance to help us make the decision. With no family history of diseases treated with cord blood, it's extremely unlikely that we'll need to tap into the banked stem cells. There's also no guarantee that the banked cord blood will be effective, should a family member ever need to use it. But there are ongoing medical trials that are promising.

If you choose to use private cord blood banking, it will run you anywhere from $1,000 to $2,000, and then there's an annual fee of approximately $125+ a year (look into discounts). Some banks may even cover the fee assessed for the doctor's collection. When investigating your options, make sure you know how the blood will be collected, the costs involved, whether you can transfer the cells from one bank to another bank, and what happens should the company go out of business.

3. DONATE IT TO A PUBLIC CORD BLOOD BANK

Public banking is free and an option that everyone should consider (ask your caregiver or contact the hospital where you'll be delivering for locations). When you donate to a public cord blood bank, the stem cells collected become available to anyone who might need them. This means that should *you* ever need your stem cells, they might not be available. Still, according to the research available, there's a reasonable chance you'll find a match in a public bank.

Donating cord blood to a public bank is relatively easy—as long as you start looking into it before the 34th week of the pregnancy and talk to your doctor or midwife. You will also need to answer screening questions. Not everyone will be eligible to donate. You can visit the National Marrow Program website (www.marrow .org) for more information. The National Marrow Donor Registry provides patients with "access to more than 11 million donors and cord blood units around the world." When you visit the website, you'll find information that walks you through how and where to donate. You can also contact them in the United States toll-free: (800) MARROW2 (1-800-627-7692). Outside the United States, call (612) 627-5800 and once connected, dial 0 for the operator.

The collection process for donating to a public cord blood bank is similar to the process when banking privately. The main difference is that once it's collected, anyone will have access to your cord blood donation.

THE BOTTOM LINE:

Whether you do it privately or publicly, bank your cord blood. It's too valuable to throw away.

Tip #78
THE PEDIATRICIAN: The Doctor Will See Your Baby Now

THE TIP:

Not all women will interview the doctor.

THE STORY:

As a teacher, I know that nothing can truly prepare you for the classroom—you just have to wait until you're there. That's how I felt about the pediatrician. Nothing I can observe in an interview can show me; it was more about what I saw once the doctor was interacting with my son. I asked all my friends who they had gone to and what they experienced. I asked the parents of students in my class. When we filled out the hospital forms, we had to list a doctor. The doctor I listed didn't end up being the doctor we used. The original doctor wasn't available to meet my son in the hospital, so another doctor from the practice came in. I had never met her before. We had an instant connection. I was having problems with breastfeeding and she was like my coach. While she wasn't taking on more patients, she made an exception for us. And that's how we found our doctor.

—Leslie, son, twenty-two months

✳✳✳

I had no idea that we had to find a doctor for the baby before the baby was born. The thought never entered my mind until my wife said, "We need to find a doctor for the baby." That's when I realized we had to find a doctor for a kid that isn't even here yet.

It's strange to get a doctor for an unborn child. The paternal instincts hadn't quite kicked in for me at that point. So finding a doctor meant having to imagine what it would be like to be a father. And that's virtually impossible because until you're a father, you can't know what it feels like.

When the baby is born, the pediatrician (or family doctor) will come to the hospital or birthing facility and examine the baby. We were required to fill out paperwork during pre-registration and list our pediatrician. So the decision needs to be made before the baby is born. A lot of women take the lead on this one (must be the maternal instincts). Had I known a little more about what to ask and what to look for, I probably could have been more supportive, but it was all foreign to me.

When interviewing your doctor, inquire about circumcision. If you decide to have your child circumcised, will the pediatrician do it, the obstetrician, or a mohel (if having a bris)?

—Chris, son, two weeks

Some people interview doctors and some use word

WANT TO SEE IF YOUR DOCTOR'S CERTIFIED?
Visit the American Board of Medical Specialties at www.abms.org.

of mouth to find the best doctor. However you and your partner approach this one, here are questions to help you figure out the best fit for your personality. One more thing I wish someone had told me—see a specialist and get a second opinion when dealing with major medical issues. Don't wait for your pediatrician to recommend it.

QUESTIONS TO ASK IN ORDER TO FIND THE RIGHT FIT

DOCTOR'S TRAINING:

- How long has the doctor been practicing?
- Where did he or she go to school?
- What are his or her particular specialties?

DOCTOR'S PERSONALITY:

- Why did he or she choose to become a doctor?
- Does he or she have kids of his/her own?
- Favorite part of the job?
- Least favorite part of the job?
- The biggest mistake new parents make?
- The thing new parents do best?

DOCTOR'S PHILOSOPHY:

- Thoughts about breastfeeding?
- Thoughts about formula feeding?
- Thoughts about immunizations?
- Thoughts about the family bed (see Tip #97)?
- Thoughts regarding circumcision?

DOCTOR'S OFFICE SERVICES:

- What are regular office hours?
- Are there weekend hours?
- When are sick appointments scheduled?
- When is well-care scheduled? What is the schedule for newborns?
- Is there a separate waiting area for sick kids (so that well and sick kids aren't intermingled)?
- How long does it take to get an appointment (emergency or non)?
- Will you always see the same doctor?
- How long are well-care appointments?
- How long are sick-care appointments?
- Does the doctor generally run on time?
- Does the doctor have a specific "phone-in hour" to answer calls?
- How long does it take to get a return call during regular office hours?
- What is the policy regarding after-hours calls? Who calls back? How long does it take to get a call back? Is there a fee?

PAYING FOR CARE:

- Is the doctor part of your insurance plan?
- Do they accept credit cards?
- Cancellation policy?

QUESTIONS FOR YOURSELF:

- Is the location convenient?
- Is parking easy?
- Is the size of the practice too big for you? Too small?
- What do other parents say?
- Most importantly, do you get a good feeling from the doctor? Is this someone you feel comfortable talking to?

THE BOTTOM LINE:

Some pediatricians charge to give medical advice after hours. Find out before calling after hours.

Tip #79
MANAGING HER PAIN: Ouch, That Doesn't Hurt

THE TIP:

When discussing your birth plan with the doctor, the part about the pain medication is her decision.

THE STORY:

It was the "labor talk," and the doctor was asking me what my plan was regarding pain medication. Obviously, for me it was no question. I already knew I was going to have

> We had to leave the room for about fifteen minutes when they did the epidural. She was looking pretty groggy at the time when I left with her mom. When we came back, she was all perky and high.
>
> —*Chris, son, twenty months*

an epidural. When the doctor asked what I planned to do, my husband chimed in and said, "Is it necessary to get an epidural? Because I've had cavities filled without Novocain before." The doctor explained that it's not the same thing. Then my husband continued to describe his experience and question my need for medication. He was totally serious about it too. The doctor explained that he didn't think anyone who's not a woman can know the experience and understand the feelings. I just looked at my husband and said, "You're f**kin' crazy. I'm getting an epidural." Once the baby was born and he saw me go through twelve hours of contractions before getting to the hospital, he realized how stupid he was to say that. I think he was just trying to be a tough guy.

—*Grace, son, two and a half*

***

> I delivered all three of our children totally naturally, and it brought my husband to tears after our first was born. He just kept telling me how incredibly strong I was.
>
> —*Cathy, sons, ten months and three, daughter, four and a half*

Until a man can deliver a seven-and-a-half-pound baby through his penis, this one is her call.

If your idea of pain relief and her idea of pain relief don't match up, she wins. When it comes to pain management during labor and delivery, women have strong feelings one way or the other. It's either "Hell yeah!" or "Hell no!" But it's something that needs to be talked about and included in the birth plan (see the box at the end of this tip for the most common pain management options).

HELL YEAH—GIVE ME THE EPIDURAL

One of the most talked-about forms of pain management is the epidural. The epidural block is administered through a flexible tube inserted into the back near the spinal cord. The procedure takes about twenty minutes. The medication can take up to twenty minutes to kick in. If administered too late, it can be ineffective. My wife was aware of this and made sure she got the epidural early into active labor (no way was she missing the pain med window). Once her contractions started to get painful, she called in the anesthesiologist and asked him to deliver the goods. He was her new best friend.

Here's how our epidural went down. The anesthesiologist asked me to leave the room during the fifteen-minute procedure. Once the meds kicked in, she was so damn happy. While the epidural numbed the pain, she could still feel the pressure of the contractions and the

> My wife had three great successful natural births without epidurals. The first one was much longer and harder. The second was quicker and easier. The third was quickest and easiest. The end of the deliveries sucked for her, but she never considered medication. She has a lot of knowledge when it comes to birth and we believe there's less risk of intervention with a natural birth.
>
> —Harell, daughters, five and three, son, two weeks

baby passing through the birth canal. (Some women have a harder time feeling the contractions while on medication.)

Of course, with any procedure, there are risks, but that's something you should discuss with your caregiver and the anesthesiologist. Whatever she chooses, it's helpful for you to have an idea of what you can do to help. This is where birthing classes, breathing, labor positions, back massages, and other techniques come in.

HELL NO—NO PAIN MEDS FOR ME

If your partner is opting for a natural birth, this doesn't mean a vaginal birth. A natural birth actually means a birth with as little medical intervention as possible. In a perfect world, for her this would mean no pain meds, no meds to induce labor, no IV (this can restrict movement), and several other criteria discussed in your birthing class. Basically, her body dictates how labor progresses—not the caregiver. Many women who plan on having a natural birth feel strongly about *not* administering medication. The problem is that never having had a baby, and never having experienced labor, it's hard to know what she will feel and what she will want until she gets there.

Make sure you know what she wants, but let her know that what she wants might change and you support her decision. After thirty-six hours of labor, she might change her mind. After ten minutes, she might change her mind. Avoid telling her to suck it up or pressuring her to work through the pain if she wants pain meds. Listen to her. If you're unsure if she's just complaining or not saying what she really feels, create a signal ahead of time that will indicate to you that she *really* wants meds. It can be some kind of code like, "Medicate me, you bitch!" Or it can be a hand gesture, like waving her middle fingers on both hands in concentric circles. It can be a physical action, like slapping your cheek. Or it can simply be, "Pain medication, please." If she has a doula or a midwife, make sure she knows the birth plan. Having it in writing helps clear up any confusion.

Whatever happens, support her decision. The *most* important thing is that the baby is healthy and that mom is healthy. The problem is that women who want a natural delivery and change their plan mid-labor have been known to feel a deep sense of guilt. A healthy baby is nothing to feel guilty about. Changing her plan should be part of the plan.

THE BOTTOM LINE:

It really doesn't hurt (they're just being dramatic). And NO, I'm not serious.

PAIN MANAGEMENT OPTIONS

Epidural Anesthesia

A doctor injects medicine into the lower part of the backbone or spine. The medicine blocks pain in the parts of the body below the shot. During a contraction, the feeling of pain travels from the uterus to the brain along nerves in the backbone. Epidurals block the pain of contractions by numbing these nerves.

Epidurals allow most women to be awake and alert with very little pain. Many women who get epidurals do not feel any pain during contractions. Medicines used in epidurals include Novocain-like drugs that block the pain in that region combined with opioids like fentanyl.

Some disadvantages of an epidural include the following:

- It can make her shiver.
- It can lower her blood pressure.
- It can make her feel very itchy.
- It can cause headaches.
- It may not numb the entire painful area, so some women continue to feel pain in the abdomen and back.

Intravenous or Intramuscular Analgesic

Pain medicine is administered through a tube inserted in a vein (intravenous) or by injecting the medicine into a muscle (intramuscular). These medicines go into the blood and help ease the pain. Opioids including morphine, fentanyl, and nalbuphine are usually used for this type of pain relief. This option does not get rid of all the pain. Instead, it usually just makes the pain bearable. After getting this kind of pain relief, a woman can still get an epidural or spinal pain relief later.

Some disadvantages of getting intravenous or intramuscular analgesics include the following:

- They make her feel sleepy and drowsy.
- They can cause nausea and vomiting.
- They can make her feel very itchy.
- These medicines cross into the baby's bloodstream and can affect the baby's breathing and heart rate and cause him/her to be very sleepy after birth.

Pudendal Block

A doctor injects numbing medicine into the vagina and a nearby nerve called the pudendal nerve. This nerve carries sensation to the lower part of the vagina and vulva. This is only used late in labor, usually right before the baby's head comes out. With a pudendal block, she has some pain relief but remains awake, alert, and able to push the baby out. The baby is not affected by this medicine, and it has very few disadvantages.

Spinal Anesthesia

A doctor injects a medicine into the lower part of the backbone. This medicine numbs the body below where the medicine was injected. Spinal anesthesia gives immediate pain relief, so it is often used for women who need an emergency C-section. Spinal anesthesia uses numbing medicines similar to Novocain combined with opioids like fentanyl.

Some disadvantages of spinal anesthesia include the following:

- It numbs the body from the chest down to the feet.
- It makes her feel short of breath.
- It can lower her blood pressure.
- It can cause headaches.

(Source: WomensHealth.gov)

Tip #80
YOU RUN THE SHOW: You Are Her Eyes, Ears, and Voice

THE TIP:

If something doesn't feel right, let someone know. Don't let anyone else run the show. You need to do what you feel is right.

> Be prepared in case the birth plan cannot be followed. It was completely stressful changing up the plan at the last minute due to complications. All that mattered at the time was the health and safety of mom and baby.
>
> —*Fred, daughter, two, sixteen weeks pregnant*

THE STORY:

The labor and delivery went along as well as could have been planned. I wasn't concerned, but the nurse and the doctor said the placenta was very large. Once the labor and delivery was complete, the nurse felt my wife's abdomen during recovery. She

- Be friendly during shift changes.
- Know where the nurse's station is.
- Know how to page for help.
- Be kind and courteous when meeting the team.
- Show everyone the birth plan (write it out).
- Listen to your partner when she needs something.
- Listen to your instincts when you need something.
- If you have questions, always ask them.
- If you don't get an answer, ask again.
- July is the season for new residents—ask to speak to an attending physician.

said it felt like her bladder was full and asked her to go to the bathroom. In hindsight, this seemed unusual because she had a catheter which had emptied the bladder. There was a good amount of blood, but no one thought that was unusual because the catheter had just been removed, and blood is part of labor and delivery. Again, in hindsight, I would have asked the doctor to feel if the uterus was contracting properly. About an hour or two later, we moved from the labor and delivery room into the hospital room. When the nurse felt my wife's abdomen, she noticed that my wife was bleeding and had soaked through a pad. The nurse changed the pad which started soaking through again. That's when I told her to call the doctor. She wanted to wait and see how things progressed. I insisted that we should call the doctor. She then called the chief resident. When the resident arrived, she noticed there was a lot of hemorrhaging. Everything moved very fast, but a hemorrhage cart was brought into the room, and there was a lot of blood. They scraped out the uterus so that the uterus could contract and stop bleeding. She was lucky enough not to need blood.

—*Mike, son, nine months, daughters, five and seven*

***

You are your partner's and your newborn's advocate. If the birth plan is the blueprint for the job, you're the foreman. You are the one to make sure that everything goes according to plan. Given that your partner will be busy during labor, you're going to be her eyes, ears, and voice. Even if a doula or midwife is assisting, you still need to be involved in the process.

It's hard to be in charge when so much of this process is new and unfamiliar. This is the reason why birthing classes and conversations with other guys who have been there (not to mention a book like this) can be helpful.

One thing about being an advocate: it can be uncomfortable at times. You might be annoying. You might disrupt the caregiver's routine. Not everyone will be patient with you. Someone might snap. Someone might get short with you. Not everyone will respond to you the way you want them to respond. That said, the majority of the medical team will be happy to address your and your partner's needs.

One way to get the medical support team on your side is to acknowledge them when you meet them. Introduce yourself. Ask how they're doing. Stop for one second

PREGNANCY Q & A

QUESTION: Most helpful thing your man did during delivery?

ANSWER: This was our second child and he's a surgery resident. The anesthesiologist didn't arrive until forty-five minutes after I asked for medication—I desperately needed the epidural. My husband found the guy and told him, "That's my wife in there and if you don't come and give her that shot, I will." —Cathy, sons, four months and three and a half

and let them know how much you appreciate them. Explain that you're a first-time father. Let them know that you might have questions and that you appreciate their patience. Start a relationship with them. Share the birth plan with them (another reason why having it in writing is useful). They will be the most important people during the birth—second to your pregnant partner. Share snacks with them. Offer them a drink when you run down to the cafeteria (not a scotch, a Diet Coke). Show them that you appreciate and value their time and services. Give 'em a little love—that's it.

Appreciate that shifts will change and, most likely, the nurses you meet when you are admitted will not be the same nurses who are there when your baby arrives. Whenever there is a shift change, make an effort to be as nice as you were the first time around. This can get hard as you get tired and the labor intensifies, but as an advocate, you need to do whatever you can to have a relationship with the people who will be in charge of her care. Share your birth plan with whoever takes over.

NOT EVERYONE WILL RESPOND

Most medical professionals do *not* make mistakes, but some do. When you play the role of a vocal, caring, and educated partner, it means asking questions—but not all caregivers want to give you attention. *Never* hold back from asking questions. When a nurse comes in and injects something into your partner or baby, ask what's being injected before the liquid flows. If the fetal monitor seems to be out of position or you're unsure of what the lines mean, ask. If the heartbeat seems too fast or too slow, say something. If something is beeping, page a nurse and find out why. Ask them to double-check dosages when administering medication to your partner or the baby. When the doctor checks her cervix to determine her progress, ask him what's happening and to explain if you don't understand. As an advocate, you have a right to know. If you're thinking it, ask about it.

THE BOTTOM LINE:

Kiss up to the nurses, but don't kiss them (not cool while your partner is giving birth).

Tip #81
GETTING IT TO COME OUT: Walking It Out and Sexing It Out

THE TIP:

Even "Dance Dance Revolution" won't get it out.

THE STORY:

Today is my due date and I've been trying to meet my

baby for the past two weeks. I've made a point to walk to the train every day during my commute. When I get to work, I'm upright and active. Last week I had a prenatal massage by someone trained in acupressure. She worked

> I asked the baby to come out on a Friday so we could have the weekend, and on Friday afternoon she went into labor. He was born Saturday. The baby heard me.
>
> —*Steve, son, nine months*

the pressure points in my ankles and feet for a good hour, but it didn't work. This past weekend, a friend of ours got the Wii. We played "Dance Dance Revolution" for a good hour. When that didn't work, I played Wii tennis for a half hour. It didn't hold my attention. We walked around the mall a couple times and still nothing. I've continued taking my prenatal yoga classes (that's supposed to help). Today I cooked a lot, thinking that being upright would help. All I have is a freezer packed full of food, but still no baby. I'm coming to terms with the fact that I have no control. I have to be patient and wait it out. The anticipation is so hard.

—*Amy, forty weeks pregnant*

✳✳✳

There will be a point when she wants it out. She will be cooked, done, finished—like when the red popper sticks out of the turkey. She will run out of patience. She will be unable to sleep, unable to hold her pee, and she will be all-around completely 100 percent done. Even the

> Lots of sex didn't work, but trying to "loosen the seal" was fun anyway.
>
> —*Patrick, expecting number six*

happiest pregnant women will sour when their due dates have come and gone and the pounds keep packing on.

How labor begins is something that science hasn't quite figured out. We have been able to create a drug that can start contractions and induce labor (Pitocin), but we don't know how to make it happen naturally. Other than a C-section or induction, it's just a waiting game.

Over the years, pregnant women have tried a number of things to induce labor—having sex, walking for hours, exercising, stimulating the nipples, eating spicy foods, drinking tea, eating pineapple, applying pressure to the ankles, acupuncture, and fasting are only some of the old wives' tales you'll hear about (interesting how they're never "young wives' tales").

Talking the baby out, walking it out, and sexing it out are some of the techniques I would suggest. Should your doctor give you the okay to have sex during the final days of the pregnancy (not all of you will get the green light), go at it. It is said that semen has a similar make-up to Pitocin (it's science, not BS). When she suspects you of trying to trick her into having sex with you, read this paragraph to her. If this isn't enough proof, Google "semen inducing labor." But before you get too excited about having sex, understand that extremely pregnant sex isn't always hot sex. I mean, it's hot if the air conditioning is broken and you're having pregnant sex in Florida in August, but don't expect it to rank in your top ten encounters. Still, any sex

> We tried everything—sex, scrubbing the floor, going for walks (which is healthy anyway so do that), spicy food…*None of it works!*
>
> —*Molly, son, four months*

you can have before she goes into her sex hibernation is good sex.

Warning: If she's approaching her due date and has yet to give birth, friends and family will call and ask if she's close. She's likely to get

> Pregnant sex is more work than it is fun. Toward the end, I just want my cervix to soften so I don't even care if I orgasm as long as I get the juices.
>
> —Jessica, daughter, three, thirty-six weeks pregnant

annoyed with everyone asking her the same question. All she wants to do is *not* think about the fact that she's *not* in labor. Having people call will just be a reminder of what she's trying to forget. You will act as the buffer for these calls. If you get tired of being a buffer, a lighthearted effective way of protecting your pregnant partner is to create a special outgoing voice mail message. You can follow the script I've provided or any variation:

> *"Hi, this is (insert your name). We're not here right now to take your call. It's not because (insert her name) is in labor, but because we're trying to go into labor. This means we're either walking around a mall or having sex. When we're back from the mall or done having sex, we'll call you back. Thanks!*

THE BOTTOM LINE:

Remind her that having sex with her is NOT for you; it's all for her.

12

THE BIRTH DAY

From Your Door to Delivery Room and Back Again

Tip #82
GOING INTO LABOR: Driving Like a Maniac and Hoping for a Room

THE TIP:
When she goes into labor, your nesting instincts will kick in. And that can mean feeling like an idiot.

THE STORY:
Being half-asleep and half in disbelief, I muttered something unintelligible like "Mhhhwahhh?" She then told me that she had been using the bathroom when all of a sudden, a gush of liquid came out. And since it was still leaking out

of her, either her water had broken or she was having the world's longest "accident." To be honest, until we got to the hospital, it didn't fully hit me that her water had broken. Or if it did, that this meant the baby was going to be delivered. But either way,

> I heard my wife screaming at 7:30 a.m. about water. We had a leaky toilet the night before. So I grabbed a plunger and towels and ran upstairs. She laughed at me and asked how I was going to deliver the baby with that.
> —*Jeff, father of two*

we needed to get to the hospital, so I sprang into action—which meant acting like an idiot. We didn't have a bag packed yet, so my wife calmly began packing while I got dressed and began pacing back and forth, unsure of what to do with myself. I kept asking her over and over if I should wear a baseball cap until I realized that I was, for some reason, asking a woman going into labor to focus her attention on whether I wore a hat.

—*Peter, son, six months*

***

The moment she starts going into labor is the moment you realize she's going to have a baby today (or tomorrow). It's real. Even after nearly forty weeks of pregnancy, until she starts going into labor, it's not real. She's known this for months, but then this thing has been kicking her every day to remind her. Once the moment hits, we realize

> I was very anxious when she went into labor. Make sure you know the route (especially if you go at night) and exactly where to park if you arrive after hours.
> —*Mike, son, twelve months*

that she needs to get to the hospital and have this baby. That can be a long, crazy, and unpredictable moment.

A man's instincts are to take her to the hospital ASAP. A woman's instincts tend to be to clean herself up—as if she's about to go to senior prom. My wife took a shower, dried her hair, and had a pedicure the day before. I started to get jealous of the doctor—she rarely got so dressed up for me. While she got prepped, I sat there in a state of shock, thinking, "Holy shit, I can't believe this is happening. We have to go." By the time my wife was ready to go, I had just realized I didn't put my things together. Now, she had to wait for me while I

SO MUCH TO REMEMBER

- Make sure you have gas. Women in labor do not like sitting in the car while you pump.
- Leave jewelry at home. It's too easy to lose.
- Refer to a list of things to do right before leaving. This should be a list you've already prepared. Include items like: take out garbage, adjust the thermostat, remember your pregnant partner. It's hard to think in that moment, so if you have a list, you won't have to do any thinking.

packed and went through my list. Women are allowed to do what they want, but if you delay them in any way, they get pissed off. Women in labor are *not* very patient.

Should she go into labor and should she leave you alone to pass the time while she showers and puts on makeup, it's

CALL YOUR HEALTH INSURANCE PROVIDER

Many health insurance providers require that you notify them within a specified period of time when she is admitted for delivery.

a good idea to go through the "what to pack list." It's also a good idea to have your "going to the hospital outfit" in mind. It sounds ridiculous, but this way you don't have to think about what to wear. It can be hard to think at that moment. You can also put together a list of things you need to do when you leave the house—things like taking out the garbage, lowering the heat or air conditioning, turning off the outdoor lights, unplugging anything that needs to be unplugged—all the same things you would do if you were going out of town for a few days. Writing it down in advance will help you focus.

Once you arrive at the hospital, you're not guaranteed entry. You can get rejected at the door. Unless you have a planned C-section or are being induced, there's no guarantee that they will give you a room. And even if you get a room, there's always a chance they can send you home once the doctor checks her out.

In order to get a room, she needs to be at a certain point in her labor. That point can vary based on your caregiver and how busy the facility is. But there's a reasonable

I almost got into two accidents on the way to the hospital. There was a blizzard, and a van almost ran into me. Then I was following a snow plow when it started to back up and just missed me. My wife was yelling at me the whole time.
—*Scott, daughter, nine months*

chance you might get rejected. The doctor might tell you to take a walk and come back in a few hours or in a few days. You won't know until you get there.

THE BOTTOM LINE:
She can take as much time as she wants when she goes into labor. You can't.

Tip #83
PASSING THE TIME: Eating, Drinking, Watching the Breastfeeding Channel

THE TIP:
Don't leave the delivery room when she's in labor. If you do, don't go home and clean to pass the time.

THE STORY:
My husband is a cop and one of those testosterone kind of guys. With our first child, it was hard for him to understand that I needed him. He was the type of man who didn't know what to do when I was having contractions. I don't know if it was because he was scared or nervous, but when he saw that I was in so much pain, he said that he had to leave and go clean the house. I was so pissed. I was trying to get through my labor, and he just got up and left. The doctor thought I'd be there all day long, but I had the baby three hours later. When my husband came back, my feet were already in stirrups and I was pushing. The second time around, he's much better. I told him he wasn't leaving this time.

—*Maria, daughter, two, thirty-four weeks pregnant*

***

Once you get settled into the room, there's a reasonable chance you'll do a lot of sitting, snacking (covertly), and avoiding sleep until the action heats up. Labor can be a long and slow process. It's not all huffing, puffing, and counting contractions. When things pick up, they'll move fast. But before then, it can be a slow crawl. It's like watching a baseball game between two last-place teams at the end of September. Labor can be slow—very slow.

If your partner is having a natural delivery with no pain meds, you'll be busy helping her through early labor. If your partner is taking pain medication, you may face hours of sitting and anticipating. It's exhausting to wait—physically and emotionally (but never complain that you are tired). It was hard enough sitting through the thirty-minute video at the birthing class—imagine thirty-two hours. Plan on how you'll pass the time. The

> My husband kept playing with everything in the delivery room. He was playing with the diapers, the hand sanitizer (he must have applied Purell a hundred times), the umbilical cord scissors, the cabinets—after a while, I tuned him out, but when he started playing with the lights, I lost it.
>
> —*Jodie, son, two and a half, daughter, ten months*

> I went through thirty-six hours of labor. He actually sat down in a chair and fell asleep! I screamed at him to wake up, and when he wouldn't, I threw a roll of medical tape at him. When that wouldn't wake him up, I threw a frozen bottle of water at him. It hit him right in between the eyes!
>
> —*Ashley, daughter, twelve months*

following are some things to keep in mind.

THINGS TO KEEP IN MIND WHILE PASSING THE TIME

- **Sleeping during labor:** She might sleep, but you shouldn't sleep—unless she wants you to sleep. If you do sleep, set your cell phone for thirty-minute increments. You want to be awake and aware. You don't want someone to perform a C-section while you're dreaming that she had a C-section.

- **Playing music:** Make sure to take an iPod or some CDs to play. It helps to pass the time. It's also something she'll enjoy focusing on when the labor gets intense. Check ahead of time if the facility has a music player.
- **Eating and drinking:** You need to eat and stay hydrated. Do your eating and drinking outside the room. If the food smells, do it far enough away where she can't smell the fries. Pack nonsmelling snacks like energy bars, trail mix, and nuts—even if Cheetos is sponsoring the birth (see Tip #66).
- **Cell phone/texting:** Women in labor don't like it when guys are on their cell phones talking about their

fantasy baseball draft. You might be nervous or anxious, but don't sit there talking on the phone. Use it sparingly. If someone calls for her, don't hand her the phone without her okay.

- **Watching TV and movies:** *SportsCenter* might be soothing for you, but not for her. If you happen to come across the breastfeeding channel, don't stay on it for too long. If she has a favorite TV show, buy the full-season DVD set and bring it along. You can also bring movies to play on your DVD or computer (again, her choice).

- **Visitors and guests:** While you might not have planned to have friends or family in the delivery room, it's nice to have other people in the mix to spice things up (if she says yes, of course). Just make sure they know that when things start moving, they will have to move back to their waiting room seats.

- **Smoking:** If you step outside for a smoke, don't bring the stink back in with you. That might disgust her. Better yet, if you do smoke, just don't smoke while she's in labor.

> When my wife was admitted, the nurse walked in and introduced herself. Then she looked at me and shouted JON. I recognized her too. She had been my boss ten years ago when we both worked together in a museum. It was a perfect fit. When I'm stressed, I talk and talk and talk. When my wife is stressed, she likes peace and quiet. So during the long waiting times, I caught up with my old coworker, and my wife got to avoid me talking her ear off. We both got what we needed.
>
> —Jon, son, three, thirty-three weeks pregnant

- **Don't be funny:** My wife told me that there's no room for joking during the labor. I thought she was joking. It turns out that she was serious. Once the epidural took hold, she appreciated the joking.
- **Seat fillers:** Like having a seat filler at the Academy Awards, if you need a break, get a stand-in. Find a family member to take your place while you run out for a snack or head to the cafeteria.
- **Leaving:** Do not leave her for long periods of time. She will need you there.
- **Working:** Do not bring work to the labor room. She wants your full attention.
- **Expelling gas:** Leave the room when you get the urge. If anything, do a tester in the bathroom to see if your gas smells. If it doesn't smell, then feel free to let it go. Otherwise, be kind and hold it in.

THE BOTTOM LINE:

Things will go from 1 mile per hour to 100 miles per hour in an instant. Be prepared for the wildest ride of your life.

Tip #84
THE BIRTH: Stage 1—Early Labor, Active Labor, Transition; Stage 2—The Birth; Stage 3—Afterbirth

THE TIP:
It might be fast and easy—easier than anyone anticipated.

THE STORY:
At 8:00 a.m., I thought I was in false labor. At 9:00 a.m.,

we started timing the contractions. At 10:00 a.m., we called the doctor and were told to go to the hospital. At 10:15 a.m., my water broke. It was kind of a trickle, and then with each contraction, it increased. My husband was driving and timing the contractions. When we got there, they said that today was the day! At 1:30 p.m., they moved me into the delivery room, and at 2:15 p.m., I got an epidural. I was really glad—I had been having contractions since 8:30 a.m., and the pain was starting to get intense. When I got the epidural, they checked me and said I was 6 centimeters dilated (they only checked me three times, because my water had broken and they didn't want to risk an infection). They told me to wait until 6:00 p.m. to start pushing because I was strep B positive, so they wanted me to have some medication beforehand. At 6:00 p.m., they said it was time to push. He came out fourteen minutes later. There was no tearing and no episiotomy; everything went well!

—*Kate, son, two weeks*

THE TIP:
It might be long and hard, but it will be worth it.

THE STORY:
We had been at the hospital for several hours before the pushing began—in fact, this was our second time there since we'd come in the night before with a "false alarm." Once the pushing began at about 9:00 p.m., it kept going for three hours. We were getting pretty tired, frustrated, and disappointed by the third hour. Our nurse kept giving us false hope by saying "good push," when in fact there was little progress. It was her way of cheering us on, but

we just wanted the truth. After about two and a half hours of pushing and twenty-four hours of labor, we said to each other that we would just do a C-section if that's what it's going to take. My wife was tired, and she was feeling claustrophobic from wearing an oxygen mask. It wasn't ideal but seemed at the time to be a better scenario than pushing for another thirty minutes with no results. Finally the doctor came in, and along with a new nurse (who took over for the previous nurse a few minutes prior), helped us make some progress on the pushing, but determined that the head was too big for the cervix (the opening was too small) to make this work. That's when the idea of the vacuum came up. We were all for it—beats a C-section for sure. We had no fears. We were aware that we'd end up with a temporary conehead, but we just wanted the baby already. We didn't have an option between vacuum and forceps. We'd been told that the doctors will use whatever they are most comfortable with. When they started preparing the vacuum, they called in a few assistants from the NICU. That made us a little nervous because it indicated something could go wrong. After two pushes and five minutes later, our little coneheaded daughter came out. I don't remember much of anything. But once I saw the head, I turned to my wife and said, "Holy shit!" The bump on her head (I always called it a brioche because it was shaped like the little knob on the top of brioche bread) was gone within a few days.

—*Jason, daughter, five months*

***

Welcome to labor and delivery.

Most men think of themselves as vagina experts, but few of us know much about labor and delivery. As the third trimester progresses, you'll hear a lot about the cervix, dilation, effacement, episiotomies, epidurals, natural birth, cesarean sections, crowning, pushing, and the placenta. I wasn't always sure what the doctors were talking about. Here's a quick summary of what's going to happen during labor and delivery and some insight into the terminology.

> The doctor wasn't there yet, just the nurse. The nurse told her to stop pushing, but my wife is like, "I gotta get this thing out of there!" I had one leg and her mom had the other leg. She was all out pushing at this point. The nurse commented that she had never seen a first-time birth go that quickly.
>
> —Bob, son, seventeen months

Imagine that the vagina is a road (call it Vagina Lane); a block or so up Vagina Lane is the cervix. The cervix is the opening to the uterus. Before getting pregnant, the uterus is the size of a pear. During pregnancy, the uterus grows to about a thousand times its original size. Now, think of a pregnant woman's uterus as a big balloon. The opening of the balloon is the cervix. For the past thirty-eight weeks, the cervix has thickened, remained closed, and been sealed off with a mucous plug (as added protection). This is why you have been able to have sex without harming the baby. The balloon holding the baby has been sealed.

The first stage of labor is when the cervix dilates or opens up (10 centimeters is fully dilated) and thins out (this is called effacement) so the baby can exit the uterus and enter the birth canal (aka Vagina Lane).

The second stage is when the baby enters the birth canal and is pushed out into the world. If the baby is too big to pass through the birth canal, a doctor might perform an epi-siotomy (cutting the skin between the vagina and the anus). The doctor might have to perform a C-section (detour). Once the baby is delivered, there's another stage.

The third and final stage of labor is the delivery of the placenta. The placenta is the organ that formed in the uterus through which the baby received nourishment from the mother. The umbilical cord is attached to the placenta. In some cultures, people will actually save and cook placenta and eat it (we didn't eat it).

STAGE 1: THE THREE PHASES

1. Early labor
2. Active labor
3. Transition

I was induced the first time, told I wasn't making progress (zero centimeters!) in the first four hours of horrendous contractions. The doctor told me I was going to have a C-section if I didn't progress in the next half hour. I told him to get the "F" out of my room and give himself an F-ing C-section.

—Amanda, expecting number five

Early labor: The earliest signs of labor (a fitting name). Contractions become regular and uncomfortable (for her, not you); the cervix begins to dilate, assuming it hasn't already started. Contractions during early labor are generally five to ten minutes apart. Early labor can last days. Usually there is plenty of time to get to your caregiver. (I'm not a betting man, but I would bet $100 that everyone reading this will make it to the hospital or birthing center before giving birth. That's how rare it is to *not* make it to your destination.) Your healthcare provider will tell you when it's time to go to the hospital.

Active labor: This is when the real action starts. Contractions become more frequent and more intense (two to four minutes apart). The cervix goes from 3 centimeters to 7 centimeters during active labor. During active labor, the lessons from the birthing class start coming into play. You can begin to help with breathing, massaging her back, playing music, counting the timing of each contraction, suggesting birthing positions, helping her find a focal point, or staying far away (if she doesn't want you that close to her).

Transition: This is the fast and furious phase. The cervix will be completely dilated and effaced. Contractions can last a minute or longer. Some women get nauseous and might vomit during this phase. As the contractions increase with intensity, everyone will assume their positions. When my wife transitioned, the room did too. The bottom third of the bed was removed and the doctor and nurse assumed the position. It all moves very quickly. When she starts to transition, stay focused on being there for her. This is when you might encounter some serious verbal abuse—and no, don't answer her back. Just listen and take it like a man helping his partner through labor.

> I was shocked when they told me to grab her leg. I thought, "Isn't there a nurse to do that?" Or at least someone who is getting paid to be there. After all, I'm paying ten grand to the hospital; I shouldn't have to hold anything.
>
> —*AJ, son, eighteen months*

> I felt like I had zero choice about cutting the umbilical cord. I initially declined, and said, "No, thanks," about three times, and then two nurses forced the skin scissors in my hand to cut.
>
> —*Todd, son, four months*

STAGE 2: THE BIRTH

It's time. The moment has arrived. Drum roll please...

The nurse told to me to grab a leg (my wife's, not the nurse's). My job was to hold her right leg (even though I'm a lefty) and help her through the contractions. Helping meant counting the seconds during each contraction. I would tell her when each contraction was building, peaking, and ending. I followed the nurse's lead. We'd tell her, "Here comes another one, it's starting, get ready, push, okay, halfway through it, almost done, a little longer, okay, relax now...you're doing great..." Because she was hooked up to a monitor, I could see the contractions build, peak, and diminish on screen. Each contraction looked like a mountain on the monitor—building, building, peaking, and descending. She would rest between each contraction (about a minute or so). This part of the process is different for every couple. Every caregiver also has his or her own style of helping her through it.

During the birthing phase, the baby moves down the birth canal. Pushing can be long, tiring, and arduous. It can last for several minutes or several hours; labor typically lasts the longest with the first child (it's not nearly as long the second or third time).

As your pregnant partner pushes, the baby's head will start crowning. This is when the top of the head is visible through the vagina. Crowning is a surreal image. Words can't describe it (so I won't even try). She'll push and then stop pushing, and a little bit of the baby's head will be

THE ELECTRONIC FETAL MONITOR

During active labor, the baby's heart rate and your partner's contractions will be tracked through the use of an electronic fetal monitor. It works by placing two electronic disks (transducers) on her belly (elastic bands wrap around her torso to hold them in place). If experiencing a natural delivery (i.e., no pain medication), an electronic fetal monitor may not be used because it restricts movement. If having an epidural, a monitor will be in use throughout the labor.

visible each time. This will be the first time you see the baby. Some guys don't want to look in that area. Personally, I was locked in on the image and in awe. I thought it was amazing, strange, and riveting. (I'll get to this more in Tip #87: Preg-Man-See, but seeing it was profound in the best way.) At one point, my daughter's head was completely out, but she was still one push away from being completely out. My wife looked down and said, "The baby looks like my brother." We didn't know if "it" was a boy or girl yet. I didn't see the family resemblance, but I didn't feel that was the time to discuss this with her. If your partner wants to look, make sure there's a mirror positioned so she can see the action (bring this up with the nurses before pushing and put it in your birth plan). For some women, seeing the movement while pushing helps them concentrate and push better.

During the birth, you'll find out if the baby can fit through the birth canal. Sometimes the baby could be turned too far in one direction or be in the breech position (with the baby's buttocks or feet first). Sometimes the birth canal can be too narrow. The umbilical cord could be in a delicate position. Until she reaches the pushing part, you won't know. If you want to know what the pushing feels like, it's like bearing down to push out a bowel movement (but according to my wife, a hundred times harder). But whatever you do, *do not* push with your partner during the birth phase. (You'll give birth to something else.)

As you move through the birthing phase, your partner might need help with the final push. She's exhausted, hasn't eaten, and has been experiencing labor for hours; she might not be able to push any more. In some situations, forceps or a suction vacuum will be used to help with the final pushes. Your partner might need some help getting through the final stretch. If for any reason she can't push, don't make her feel bad about it. Do not pressure her. Do not force her. Do not make her feel guilty. It's exhausting—support, encourage, and listen to her.

As she is pushing, the doctor will work to make sure she doesn't have any vaginal tearing. If the baby can't make it through the birth canal without tearing, the doctor might opt to do an episiotomy. This means cutting the area between the

> They hooked up an electronic fetal monitor to my wife and the baby. When my wife pushed, the baby's heart rate went nuts. I thought the baby was in terrible danger. Apparently, when I mentioned something to the nurse, I was told that it's fairly normal.
>
> —Eric, daughter, twenty months

anus and the vagina to make more room for the baby to pass through the birth canal. Discuss with your doctor beforehand if she does not want this, but usually it's done to prevent painful tearing. Once the baby and placenta are delivered, the doctor will stitch up any cuts or tears. Once the head is out, the rest of the baby comes fast. Then, the baby is born. This is when the umbilical cord is clamped, and you get to cut (or not cut). Sometimes the doctor will insist that you cut the cord. You can say "no" if you're not comfortable. After a quick hello, the baby is taken for some cleaning and testing, and mom begins stage 3. DO NOT let them whisk the baby away if you want to spend a little time bonding. We didn't know we could control this. When my son was born, we told them to let Mom hold him first. Those first few minutes together were beyond special. We intend to do the same with our third baby. But you need to tell your doctor and nurses first. Assuming there are no complications, they'll respect your wishes.

STAGE 3: THE PLACENTA ARRIVES

Stage 3 surprised me. No one ever talks about this phase. I had no idea there was a stage 3. While everyone is celebrating the birth of the baby, the placenta (the organ attached to the other end of the umbilical cord) is still inside your partner. On one side of the room, your partner is delivering the placenta. On the other side of the room, nurses are cleaning, testing, stamping feet, and doing the Apgar test (see Tip #89).

As the one who's supposed to be there for your partner, it can be a bit confusing where you should go—do you videotape the baby? Snap photos? Or do you stick with the

ATTENTION, DADS OF PREEMIES

About 12 percent of you will experience it. If your child ends up in the NICU, you will become trained and supported to be a caregiver. Some advice from a dad who's done it twice (once at twenty-five weeks and once at twenty-eight weeks):

- Find a primary who you trust and like. He or she will be your child's strongest advocate.
- The nurses will train you to care for your child (CPR included).
- Have a physical outlet to blow off steam. It can get intense, and emotions can run wild.
- Take care of yourself and find support.
- Encourage your partner to find support.

mom and help her get over the final stage? I stuck with the baby and kept an eye on my wife. I felt like this was the right thing to do at the time, but never having talked about it, a part of me felt like I was abandoning her. I explained this to her after the delivery, but it would have been nice to have talked about this part of the process beforehand. She didn't have a problem with it, but I know other women have. Consider making a plan so that she doesn't feel like you're running off with the baby.

Once the placenta is delivered, the doctor will clean up your partner and make sure everything is as it should be. If you have a second, check out the placenta. It was the home base for baby; it's what's nourished him or her. Some people will take the placenta home and plant it in the backyard. Other people will cook it. We didn't eat it, cook it, or smoke it and turn it into placenta jerky, but I did take a picture of it. And you can see that picture at www .DadsExpectingToo.com. (Thank you to my wife for allowing me to post the picture of the placenta.)

THE BOTTOM LINE:
Stage 4: The Celebration.

Tip #85
THE C-SECTION SECTION: About One-Third of New Dads Will See It This Way

THE TIP:
It was seven minutes from the time I sat down until she was born. Had I known it would go so fast, I wouldn't have waited to pee.

THE STORY:
We weren't planning on a C-section delivery. The doctor explained to me that the labor stalled at 4 centimeters dilation. We prepped and signed the forms. By 7:30 a.m., the paperwork was done. I asked if I would be allowed in the operating room. I was told "Yes." I was then given a plastic kit with scrubs (pants, a mask, and hat). They didn't give me any instructions other than, "We'll get you when we're ready." My wife was wheeled for prep and I changed into my scrubs. All alone, I was left sitting in the labor and

delivery room by myself. I had to pee, so I went into the bathroom for a second. From 9:30 a.m. to 9:39 a.m., I sat in the room waiting—I imagined that they came to get me while I was in the bathroom, and I missed the delivery. Finally, they came for me at 9:40 a.m. By 9:42 a.m., I was standing in a brightly lit operating room looking at my wife, who was splayed out as if she was being crucified. A drape was set up a few inches below her chin so she couldn't see what was happening. I sat down in the chair next to her—also behind the drape. There was a resident to my right, the doctor on the other side, and four nurses and the anesthesiologist in the room. They told me it was going to go fast and that really soon I was going to be a dad. That's when I started to get nervous. It was hard to breathe with the mask. I kept thinking of all the stories of guys passing out, and it made me think about passing out. My heart started racing. The doctor told me, "Any minute now." I then heard them say, "Oh, look at the chubby cheeks." They told me to stand up and

said, "You have a beautiful girl." All I remember is locking in on her face and seeing them pulling her out. I was locked on her eyes. After the delivery, they took her across the room, wiped her down, weighed her, and made sure she was doing well. About five minutes later, they called me over to meet her and cut a few inches off of the umbilical cord. She was on the scale weighing in at 8 pounds, 4 ounces.

> The amount of blood that gushed out after the initial C-section incision freaked me out. It looked like so much, like we were in trouble. I later found out it wasn't all that much.
>
> —Anonymous

The nurses then wrapped her up and I carried her over to my wife. The whole time, my wife hadn't seen her. I got to see her first. That was special. I walked over to my wife and handed her our daughter. It was seven minutes from the time I sat down until she was born.

> —Anthony, daughter, two weeks

***

I was delivered via C-section before it was trendy to have a C-section. I like to think of my mom as a trendsetter.

Seriously, according to the Centers for Disease Control, 32.8 percent of all U.S. births in 2011 were delivered via C-section. Whether she's planning for a vaginal or C-section delivery, ask the doctor to walk you through the procedure. Ask if you'll be in the room the whole time. Ask if she will get to hold the

> We had two C-sections and I did not want to watch anything...I've heard others who want to watch. I think talking about those expectations WAY before getting to the hospital is important. My partner supported me in the fact I didn't want to cut the cord...
>
> —Kipp, daughters, four and one

> When the time came, the doctor said, "Okay, you can look now!" I looked over the divider to see a doctor holding a pile of guts. The other doctor said, "Oops, my bad. Not yet." Whew. That *Alien* thing was real for one second.
> —*Jim, daughter, two, son, eleven*

baby right away. Ask whatever questions are on your mind. If it's an unplanned C-section, make sure to support your partner. Be flexible and adjust your plan. Labor is unpredictable—your support of your partner needs to be unwavering.

You might be planning to have a C-section delivery. You might be planning for a vaginal birth. The reasons for the C-sections vary—some are because of medical issues, some due to the position of the baby, some due to developing situations, and some for convenience. (This way no one misses the game on TV.) Whether or not you're planning a C-section, here are some things to keep in mind:

1. An epidural or spinal block is the most common form of medication. Your partner will most likely be awake and alert during the procedure. They will also insert a catheter into her urethra (to drain urine). See Tip #79 for more on pain meds.

2. Most facilities will allow you in the operating room during the procedure. You'll scrub in and wear the appropriate clothes. If it's an emergency C-section or if your partner is under a general anesthetic (meaning she's not awake), you might not be allowed inside.

3. Once in the operating room, they will most likely position a screen to keep you from watching the early part of the procedure. If you want to see the action,

ask to have the screen lowered when the baby leaves the womb. You might be allowed to stand and see the procedure.

4. Recovery is longer than with a vaginal birth. It can be a three- or four-day hospital stay. This is major surgery, and with any major surgery, there is an increased risk of infection and other complications. Things like walking up stairs and picking up the baby should be avoided afterward.

5. A C-section isn't a reflection on a mom doing something right or wrong. If it's something that needs to happen, allow it to happen. Sometimes the cervix won't thin or dilate, or the baby is too big, or too excited, or in distress. Sometimes mom can be in distress.

THE BOTTOM LINE:

Ask your doctor to walk you through the procedure, even if it's not part of the birth plan. If there is an emergency, there won't be time to discuss it. This way, you'll be prepared.

Tip #86
THE CONEHEAD: And Other Newborn Oddities

THE TIP:
Imagine your baby's head getting squeezed out of a tiny hole. Then watch the *Coneheads* movie. That's what you should expect.

THE STORY:
I've got one of my wife's legs on my shoulder and the nurse had her other leg on her shoulder. My wife kept looking at me because the expression on my face was like, "What's going on here?" I tried to keep a straight face. After my son fully came out, I told her he had such a conehead that the money we put aside for college was going to have to go toward plastic surgery. He looked like he came straight out of the movie. Thank God, a day or two later, the conehead went down. With a hat on his head, he looked like a cute baby. Without the hat, his head was scary-looking. My daughter was smaller, and I don't think she was affected by going through the birth canal. But my son had such a big head that squeezing out made it look longer and pretty ugly. We had no expectations about how the baby would look, and the conehead shocked me.

—*Corey, son, two and a half, daughter, eight months*

✳✳✳

Getting pushed through the cervix and being forced down the birth canal is like getting pushed through a very crowded bar on New Year's Eve in Times Square.

Newborn babies are squeezed, pushed, pulled, suctioned, cut (from the cord), forcepped, and forced from a liquid world to dry land. Their lungs literally go from breathing fluid one second to breathing air the next. Their skin can be coated with a white pasty substance. They might have splotches on their skin from the ride down Vagina Lane. They might have hair in strange places. Their faces can appear swollen. Their heads are elongated.

While childbirth is absolutely beautiful, a newborn out of the womb has a look of her own—like a boxer who just went fifteen rounds. You will think the baby is beautiful, but the conehead or some other newborn vanity issue might freak you out. If the medical staff isn't worried, then don't be worried. I still have a hard time understanding how this could be normal, but coneheads are normal.

My daughter had the most elongated head I've ever seen. One time, my wife pushed and stopped while my daughter's head was halfway through the opening. The entire top of her head was pushing out like an eraser on top of a pencil. I wanted to push her head out, but pushing would have left me with other problems. After a couple more contractions and pushes, my daughter's head cleared. By this time, her head was completely elongated. I asked the doctor if this was normal. I couldn't imagine how this could be normal. The doctor explained that the baby's skull plates are soft and able to shift during delivery. The bones have yet to harden or fuse. This flexibility allows the skull to pass through the birth canal. After a few hours of relaxation, my daughter's head was looking rounder. The next day, she no longer had that conehead.

An elongated head was just one of several things no one

warned me about. When your kid makes his or her first appearance, you might be surprised that the baby doesn't look like you expected. Some things to prepare for include the following:

- The baby's skin could be covered with grayish greasy paste. This is called vernix, and it protects the baby's skin in the fluid environment. There might also be some newborn acne, red splotches, and wear and tear from birth.
- The baby's head might be misshapen and bruised. The skull plates shift during birth, allowing the head to travel safely down the birth canal. Don't worry about this hurting the brain—again, a conehead is normal.
- Your baby's eyes will look puffy. There might be broken blood vessels on the eyelids from the pushing. Eyes might have a hard time opening. Focusing on objects more than a few inches away could make the baby appear cross-eyed.
- If you have a boy, his genitals will look huge. (Yes, I know you're proud, but it's temporary.) If you have a girl, there will be swelling in the genital area too. The increase in hormones causes this to happen, and it's normal.
- The belly button has the remains of the umbilical cord hanging out (it's clipped). The cord will eventually fall off naturally (or the doctor will remove it), but it may look a little strange, especially with the clamp attached to it.
- The baby's skin color might look a little blue, yellow, red, or another shade of the rainbow. If the shade varies from your shade, ask your doctor about it. High levels of bilirubin will give the skin a jaundiced (yellow)

look; if it's really low, they might put your baby under a blue light.

THE BOTTOM LINE:
Even the most coneheaded, puffy-eyed, greasy-feeling, huge-scrotumed, hairy baby is beautiful.

Tip #87
PREG-MAN-SEE: You'll Never See Anything Like It Again (Unless You Do This Again)

THE TIP:
Get in there as much as you can, enjoy it, and expect to be surprised.

THE STORY:
During labor, I saw something my wife tried to prepare me for, but still, I wasn't prepared. I was standing over the doctor's shoulder during the heavy pushing. I wanted to see it all. She had been pushing for a good twenty minutes, and I could start to see the head come out. In the middle of one of the intense contractions, I saw a couple of pieces of poop drop out. The doctor waited until my wife finished the contraction and casually moved it to the side. To them, it was just part of doing business and no big concern. My wife told me this might happen, but it still

> Hell yes, I looked. It was amazing. The most intense and emotional experience of my life by far.
>
> —Eric, daughter, twenty-two months

surprised me. It didn't bother me though. With the level of excitement involved with the birth, it paled in comparison when all was said and done. Being there and watching the baby coming out was the most exciting moment of my entire life. I had the best seat in the house—I would definitely recommend it. The crowning moment was when my daughter came into the world. I couldn't imagine not seeing the whole thing.

—Scot, daughter, fourteen months

***

The SV (sex vagina) is what you saw when you got her pregnant. The BV (birthing vagina) is what you'll see if you watch her give birth. The two are distinctly different. This once sexual part of her body will be truly transformed into something entirely different. It's like Clark Kent changing into Superman, Robert Downey Jr. becoming Iron Man, or Toby Maguire turning into Spider-Man. The BV is NOT the SV.

The thought might freak you out—and yes, it's expected. Considering we are the first generation of dads in the delivery room, we're the ones who are seeing it for the first time. What you decide is a personal decision, but I can tell you that what you imagine you will see and what you will actually see (should you look) are entirely different.

I looked the first time. I looked the second time. And I'm going to look the third time. Each time the sight has been amazing, horrific, and beautiful all at once. I can't lie. It was freaky to see my wife's vagina all stretched out. That thing is flexible. I couldn't look away. I was riveted. The image is burned into my memory. And let me tell you, looking didn't ruin the vagina for me. If anything, it made me even more connected to it. I still love my wife and find her incredibly attractive. And just so you know, her vagina shrunk back to its original SV shape and form following the delivery (it can take several weeks).

> Yes, and I am happy that I watched it all. Why wouldn't I want to? It was a once-in-a-lifetime chance to see this, which also happens to be kind of a miracle!
>
> —Dan, son, four months

Here's why I suggest looking—what I saw and felt while watching my daughter and son being born into this world was the most powerful feeling I've ever experienced in my life. The emotions are unmatched. In retrospect, I wouldn't have wanted to look anywhere else. I've talked to guys who are just as happy they didn't look and I've talked to guys who share my sentiments. It's watching a miracle unfold before your eyes.

For me:

- Looking was *not* disgusting.
- Looking didn't scare me.
- Looking did *not* damage our sex life.

Going into labor, my wife was 100 percent sure she didn't want me to look. I didn't argue. By the time we hit transition, she was *not* focused on where I was looking. And she was looking. As labor progressed, she even used a mirror (another thing she didn't think she'd want) so she could see the pushing. The mirror was motivating because she could see her pushing progress (something I've also heard from other women). It's like having a rearview mirror, but you're not looking at the rear view. Even the way she saw her vagina changed. What she thought she was going to want and what she wanted at the time of delivery were two different things.

Until you're there, you don't know. Some guys won't look and will never look—but I say look. I didn't pass out. I didn't scream. And it was not a turnoff. If you love your partner and know what to expect, it will only make you closer.

THE BOTTOM LINE:
You've never seen anything like it in your life—I guarantee it.

Tip #88
LIGHTS, CAMERA, ACTION!: A Once-in-a-Lifetime Shot at the Perfect Shot

THE TIP:
Don't worry about cutting the cord—worry about getting the shot.

THE STORY:
There was this great shot of my son on the scale where his wiener wasn't visible. I needed to get the same shot of our second baby. When the baby came out, the doctor kept asking me if I wanted to cut the cord. I told him I didn't want

to cut it. I felt a lot of pressure to get the video, and there are missed shots that you can never get back. He asked me again. I said, "I'm trying to get a shot here. I can't cut the cord. I don't want to cut the cord. I'll be spending my life with the baby, and cutting the cord isn't as important as getting this shot." All I wanted was to get the shot. I got the shot. I also made sure to be careful what I shot. Last time, I accidentally took a picture of something I didn't realize. We load all our pictures into the computer's screensaver, which rotates through about a thousand shots. One day, we had some friends over, and I ran into the other room to get something when I saw a picture of my wife completely naked in the delivery room. I looked to see if anyone else saw it and I was safe. I deleted it so that no one ever knew. It could have been a disaster.

—*Gary, sons, eight months and three and a half*

***

The big question: does an adult man or woman really need to see a video of him- or herself exiting his mother's vagina?

Never before have there been more opportunities to capture the images of the first minutes of your baby's life. As someone who spends a lot of time videotaping family moments, I know that there's a dramatic difference between seeing something

Forget the video camera. We brought one, thinking we'd videotape the birth from some prime angle where my wife would look beautiful and you wouldn't see her persqueeter. But no such angle exists in reality.

—*Eric, son, eighteen months*

> We set a tripod and recorded her face and legs from the side to avoid a crotch shot.
> —*Jason, daughter, five months*

with my own eyes and seeing something through the lens of the camera. I'm grateful that the hospital had a policy that prohibited videotaping the actual birth. The rules allowed us to take photos and videos before and immediately following the birth, but not during it. Even if there wasn't a policy prohibiting it, I can't imagine that I'd want to do it after I thought it through.

Here are five reasons why:

1. Operating a video camera means having to concentrate on something other than her. She deserves all the attention.
2. Even if I set the camera up on a tripod on a static shot, I would have to worry about the tape, battery, graphic shots, or knocking it over.
3. Videotaping before and after the moment can capture the essence of the moment.
4. I have enough video to show at special events.
5. Some things are better left to the imagination.

If you do decide to take pictures or video, make sure you have a plan. Ask your partner what she's comfortable with. If she resists, explain that you can put this together in a scrapbook page for the baby. It's not for you; it's for him or her. When it comes to the actual birth, make sure she knows that you might have to leave her side. If you want to capture pictures of the baby being weighed, stamped, and washed, you're going to have to go to the other side of the room while she's in the midst of stage 3. The most important thing is that documenting the birth doesn't take away from her level of comfort and relaxation. Talking about it and having a plan will help avoid any accidental asshole moments on your part.

THE EQUIPMENT

If there has ever been a time to warrant shopping for electronics, this is it. Make her a deal—you'll go to Best Buy and she'll go to Babies "R" Us, and you'll meet back in two

THE RIGHT EQUIPMENT

- Consider getting a Wi-Fi digital camera. These cameras allow you to download photos without memory cards or USB cables. You point, shoot, and then send your pictures to your computer or a photo website.
- Get a bigger memory card and avoid having to be selective about the photos you want to take. Just point and shoot again and again.
- If purchasing a new video camera, consider getting one that records onto an internal hard drive that can be downloaded to your computer. Avoid having to purchase and keep track of digital videotapes. Purchase two hard drives (one to download videos to and one to back up the videos).

hours. She can pick you up. If you don't have a digital camera, consider getting one along with a memory card with huge capacity (which is inexpensive). You want the flexibility to take as many pictures as you want. With digital technology, even the worst photographer has the opportunity to take hundreds of crappy photos in search of one good one. The chances of getting that one good one are high when you take a thousand shots within a ten-minute window.

PLAN YOUR SHOOT

- Investigate the facility's policies when it comes to video and photos.
- Discuss what will happen once the baby is born. (Will you stay by her side or snap photos of the baby?)
- Ask your doctor or midwife if he or she has any requests. Make sure whatever you're doing isn't going to get in the way.

If you don't want to worry about downloading pictures or dealing with a memory card, consider getting a Wi-Fi camera. A new generation of cameras allows you to snap photos and then download them to a computer, a cellular network, or the Internet without having to remove a memory card or bring a USB cable. Once you snap the photo, you can send it within minutes.

If you don't own a video camera or want a new video camera, this is a great time to do it. The prices are inexpensive compared to even a year ago. For this next pregnancy, I'm contemplating a camera with an internal hard drive. This way, I won't have to worry about keeping track of digital videotapes and downloading them. If you have a video camera with a hard drive, you can download videos directly to your computer and to a backup hard drive. The general rule is that for every gigabyte, you get one hour of video (this can vary). As for downloading, memory prices have also decreased dramatically. You can find a 160-gigabyte hard drive for less than $100 (probably less by the time this book prints). When it comes to finding the best camera and best deal, shop around and then consider buying online (you can avoid the sales tax). Just make sure to buy from a reputable retailer that guarantees its products. Make sure your computer is compatible with your new equipment.

One more thing worth mentioning: it's also a good idea to bring your laptop with you to the hospital (if you have one). When things settle down, you can download the pictures and send them to your list of contacts. In just a few hours following the birth, you can send an email birth announcement, post the photo on your Facebook profile, or send a photo via your phone.

THE BOTTOM LINE:

If you do videotape the entire birth from all angles with tight close-ups in high definition, this could be a fantastic video to show your son's or daughter's future significant others to promote birth control.

Tip #89
WHAT HAPPENS NEXT?: Newborn Care, Crowd Control, and Sleep

THE TIP:

When the baby is born, skin-to-skin contact is the best way to bond.

THE STORY:

It was by chance that I came across kangaroo care when I was doing research on a project. Kangaroo care is based on how kangaroos use skin-to-skin contact to comfort newborns. It can be chest-to-chest or any skin-to-skin contact, and it helps regulate the baby's temperature and heart rate. It's soothing. As soon as he was in the room, I would open my shirt and lay him on my chest. It was an amazing experience and connection. He seemed to be comforted by me—it was profound that he could be comforted by me. There were so many benefits to it. When we were in the hospital, the nurses would come into the room and notice me and say, "Oh, kangaroo care!" I can't recommend it enough.

—Todd, son, three months

✳✳✳

ONCE THE BABY IS BORN

Once the baby is born, things will happen—fast.

If she has a vaginal delivery, you may be asked if you want to cut the cord. Once your child is born, the baby will be taken over to another area of the room and examined after the birth. Before the baby is examined, the mom can request to hold him or her. If you are following the Bradley Method or the Lamaze philosophy, immediate contact with the mother following delivery is encouraged. This means the moment the baby is born, skin-to-skin contact and comfort are the chosen approach. If nursing, breastfeeding as soon as possible is another component of aftercare. Whatever you and your partner want to have happen, make sure you communicate this to your doctor, midwife, and medical team. If having a C-section, ask the doctor to walk you through the aftercare before the procedure. It can vary based on the hospital.

After the birth, the doctor showed our daughter to my wife and then the nurses took the baby to another area of the room where they examined her, performed the Apgar test, cleaned her off, put a bracelet on her ankle, and stamped her feet. Since we never discussed the aftercare, we just went with the flow. But if you have preferences, you can change the flow. It's your delivery and your child.

The following are standard tests and procedures that will be conducted once your newborn arrives (source: www.womenshealth.gov). Ask your caregiver to go over the specifics; procedures can vary based on local laws and hospital procedures. If you are uncomfortable with any part of a procedure, discuss it with your caregiver.

> The family is going to be needy—people may come over too much. The hospital room is very small, and people just stand around watching you and the baby.
>
> —*Gary, sons, eight months and three and a half*

WAIT...DON'T BE SO QUICK TO CLAMP THAT CORD

Timing of Umbilical Cord Clamping After Birth (American College of Obstetricians and Gynecologists, December 2012 Statement)

The optimal timing for clamping the umbilical cord after birth has been a subject of controversy and debate. Although many randomized controlled trials in term and preterm infants have evaluated the benefits of delayed umbilical cord clamping versus immediate umbilical cord clamping, the ideal timing for cord clamping has yet to be established. Several systematic reviews have suggested that clamping the umbilical cord in all births should be delayed for at least thirty to sixty seconds, with the infant maintained at or below the level of the placenta because of the associated neonatal benefits, including increased blood volume, reduced need for blood transfusion, decreased incidence of intracranial hemorrhage in preterm infants, and lower frequency of iron deficiency anemia in term infants. Evidence exists to support delayed umbilical cord clamping in preterm infants, when feasible. The single most important clinical benefit for preterm infants is the possibility for a nearly 50 percent reduction in intraventricular hemorrhage. However, currently, evidence is insufficient to confirm or refute the potential for benefits from delayed umbilical cord clamping in term infants, especially in settings with rich resources.

Apgar Evaluation: The Apgar test is a quick way for doctors to figure out if the baby is healthy or needs extra medical care. Apgar tests are usually done twice: one minute after birth and again five minutes after birth. Doctors and nurses measure five signs of the baby's condition:

- Heart rate
- Breathing
- Activity and muscle tone
- Reflexes
- Skin color

Apgar scores range from 0 to 10. A baby who scores 7 or more is considered very healthy. But a lower score doesn't always mean there is something wrong. Perfectly healthy babies often have low Apgar scores in the first minute of life. In more than 98 percent of cases, the Apgar score reaches 7 after five minutes of life. When it does not, the baby needs medical care and close monitoring.

Eye Care: The Centers for Disease Control and Prevention (CDC) recommend that all newborns receive eye drops or ointment to prevent infections they can acquire during delivery. Sexually transmitted diseases (STDs) including gonorrhea and chlamydia are a main cause of newborn eye infections.

These infections can cause blindness when left untreated.

Silver nitrate, erythromycin, and tetracycline are the three medicines used in newborns' eyes (erythromycin is mostly used these days). These medicines can sting and/or blur the baby's vision, so you may want to talk to your caregiver for more details. Some parents question whether this treatment is really necessary. Many women at low risk for STDs do not want their newborns to receive eye medicine, but there is no evidence to suggest that this medicine harms the baby. It is important to note that even pregnant women who test negative for STDs may get an infection by the time of delivery. Plus, most women with gonorrhea and/or chlamydia don't know it because they have no symptoms. The antibiotic eye ointments may also help prevent infection with other bacteria, besides the ones that cause STDs.

Vitamin K Shot: The American Academy of Pediatrics recommends that all newborns receive a shot of vitamin K in the upper leg. Newborns usually have low levels of vitamin K in their bodies. This vitamin is necessary for blood clotting. Low levels of vitamin K can cause a rare but serious bleeding problem. Research shows that vitamin K shots prevent dangerous bleeding in newborns. Newborns probably feel pain when the shot is given, but babies don't seem to have any discomfort afterward.

Newborn Metabolic Screening: Doctors or nurses prick your baby's heel to take a tiny sample of blood. They use this blood to test for many diseases. All fifty states require testing for at least two disorders: phenylketonuria and congenital hypothyroidism. But many states test for up to thirty different diseases. All of these problems are impossible to spot without a blood test. And if left untreated, they can cause mental retardation and even death. The March of Dimes recommends that all newborns be tested for at least twenty-nine diseases, even if your state doesn't require it.

Hearing Screening: Many hospitals perform newborn hearing screenings. Tiny earphones or microphones are used to monitor how the baby reacts to sounds. Newborn hearing tests can detect hearing problems early, which can help cut the risk of serious language and speech problems. Universal hearing screening is recommended by the AAP. These tests measure brainwaves though and don't measure a baby's reaction to sound in the traditional sense.

Hepatitis B Vaccine: Most hospitals now suggest that newborns get a vaccine to protect against the hepatitis B virus (HBV). The hepatitis B vaccine is a series of three different shots. The second and last shot should be given before eighteen months of age.

MANAGING MOM'S AND BABY'S AFTERCARE

Once the baby is born, you are in charge of making sure your partner and the baby are getting the care they need. (I know you're tired and need to relax, but there's just a little more you need to do.) If you do not want the baby to undergo a particular test or procedure, tell the medical team before the birth; then, just in case, stick with the baby once it's born. The only way to ensure that the care you desire is administered is to be there while care is being administered. The only exception would be if there's an emergency. When it comes to your partner's recovery, don't be so quick to leave her and go home. See Tip #80 about being her advocate. The first twenty-four to forty-eight hours are important for you to be there to make sure she's comfortable. While chances are small that there will be complications following delivery, it's worth sticking around.

AFTER THE BABY IS BORN, THEY WILL

- Measure the newborn's weight, length, and head.
- Take the baby's temperature.
- Measure his breathing and heart rate.
- Give the baby a bath and clean the umbilical cord stump.

MANAGING THE CROWDS

Once the baby is born, people will want to come by. Your partner will be excited and exhausted—it's been a long day. Again, you are the guy working the door. The room is small, and she's going to need to rest. Also, you're going to want

If you're worried about the baby being away from you because of security reasons, ask the hospital what procedures are in place. Our hospital had a bracelet system that activated an alarm if the baby was taken out of the maternity ward.

time to get to know how the baby works and bond as a family. (Kangaroo care is great.) Doing things like changing diapers, feeding the baby, caring for the umbilical stump, burping the baby, and soothing the baby are things the nurses can help you with.

Once the baby is born, send out an email (using a list you've prepared) and share the specifics. You can briefly mention everything about the baby, "Mom is doing great—very tired, but great. I'll be in touch with more updates in the next few days." If everyone knows all is well and that she's tired, that should help to keep the calls to a minimum. When people call asking to visit, it might be a good idea to have them come by after she gets home, given that you're only in the hospital for two days and visiting hours can be limited. If people want to do something nice, suggest that they bring over lunch or dinner (if you're comfortable asking). If she wants visitors, make sure to let the visitors know that she's tired but would *never* tell them. One more thing, when you do have visitors, ask them to wash their hands when they come in, especially if they want to hold the baby. The nurses wash up; so should everyone else.

He didn't spend the night with me either time. The room was too small, it wasn't private, and I just wanted to sleep.

—*Collette, daughters, five months and five*

> I slept on the uncomfortable pullout. On the last night, they kicked our daughter out of the nursery and into our room because she was crying. We got no sleep. After the nurse kicked our daughter out of the nursery, we walked by the window and saw the empty nursery and her playing solitaire on the computer.
>
> —*David, daughter, six months*

WHERE BABY SLEEPS AT NIGHT

Where your newborn sleeps in the hospital will be a decision you need to make. Most likely, you will have the option of having the baby sleep in the room with mom (known as "rooming in") or having the baby sleep in the nursery. Although there's been a movement toward having the baby room in with Mom, don't be afraid to ask for the baby to spend time in the nursery if you want your partner to sleep and recover. If the baby is nursing (breastfeeding) and sleeping in the nursery, a nurse will bring the baby to Mom when the baby gets hungry. If the baby is bottle-fed, the mom doesn't have to do the feeding. You might want to have the baby in the room to spend the night together as a family, which makes sense. However, you will share many nights as a family at home, but you also won't have a lot of good nights' sleep or a night nurse to take care of your baby. A night nurse is a luxury. We quickly realized that the nursery was a *great* thing. Whatever your philosophy, know that you have an option. We learned that we could be loving parents and still have our daughter sleep in the nursery.

WHERE YOU SLEEP AT NIGHT

Given that fathers have historically not been an intricate part of the birthing process, many hospitals were not built to accommodate fathers spending the night with their partners following birth. If sharing a room with another patient, the father might not have the option of spending the night. Should the rules allow you to spend the night in the room, you may have to sleep on a chair, a couch, or a cot. Investigate this beforehand when selecting a birthing facility. If you do spend the night and are uncomfortable, don't tell her about it. I made the mistake of complaining. After giving birth, she doesn't want to hear you complain.

THE BOTTOM LINE:

Let the nurses help as much as possible. Don't be a hero. Once you go home, you can be a hero all night long.

Tip #90
LEAVING THE HOSPITAL: Taking Everything You Can Fit through the Door

THE TIP:

Stockpile as you go and check the supply closet door. You might just find yourself in the middle of Fort Knox.

THE STORY:

We raided the place. I even snuck into the supply room. Everyone told us we should clean out the supply cart because it will be replenished. I cleaned it out, stockpiled stuff in bags, then took it home nightly. Every morning, they would refill the cart and I would stockpile again. One time when I went to get ice, I noticed the supply room door near the kitchen. It's always under tight lock and key.

> Take extra bags and slowly fill your car with all their goodies! The nurses told me to! Take some snacks!
>
> —*Nancy, daughter, fifteen months*

I checked the door and somehow it opened. I was like "Ooooohhhhhhhhh, all this stuff." It was like raiding Fort Knox. I went to town grabbing wipes, diapers, swaddle blankets, onesies, changing pads, formula—as much formula as I could take with me. The next day, I tried the door again; they had closed it, but not before I had gotten what must have been two weeks' worth of supplies.

—*David, daughter, six months*

***

It's not shoplifting. The $20,000 hospital bill includes some stuff.

When you leave the hospital, you're going to want to take everything home that fits through the door. Do not take anything that is nailed down or needs electricity. (Do not take the nurses; that's called kidnapping.) Some supplies are meant to be taken. Even if you get charged for something you take, your insurance company might end up covering the bill as a special gift to you (also called a mistake).

> We finally get home for the first time with our son, and I realized I left the connection to the breast pump at the hospital and she needed to pump. I had to get back in my car and turn around and drive back by myself.
>
> —*Irl, son, twenty-two months, twenty-eight weeks pregnant*

Do not be shy about hoarding supplies. Hospitals

have lots of baby supplies
that are hard to find in the
outside world. Even if you
can get these items outside,
it's better to have as much
of it as possible when you
get home. Newborn shirts
that snap on the side (to
avoid rubbing the umbili-
cal stump), receiving blankets for swaddling, diapers,
diaper cream, blankets,
maxi pads, alcohol pads,
changing pads, gauze pads,
icepacks, baby bottles (the
two-ounce ones are hard to find), blankets, formula (for
now or later), and whatever else catches your eye—these
are all things you should take with you. I'm not saying to
steal anything, just take it—and if they stop you, just say,
"Oh, sorry."

One additional bit of advice for when you're hoarding
and stockpiling—ask for more (and they actually did give
us more). By the time we were ready to leave, we had three
bags' worth of supplies. We asked the nurses for more. And
five minutes later, the nurse walked in with more. Ask and
you shall receive more supplies or dirty looks.

Do not leave anything behind! Just make sure you go
through the list of what you brought and check it off as
you pack up to leave. Should you leave something behind,
there's a good chance you'll have to go back to get it. And
the last thing you're going to want to do is drive back to the

hospital after driving home. This will be especially true if you've raided the place and still somehow managed to leave something behind.

One more reminder: remember that to get out the door and in the getaway car with your stuff, you'll need an infant car seat—it's required by law. If you haven't installed the car seat by week thirty-five, do it. Usually the hospital can't help you with the installation. Make sure to follow the instructions and get it checked at a child seat fitting station. You don't want to be figuring out how to install the seat while your wife and newborn are waiting in the lobby for you to pull up in the getaway car (see Tip #64 for information on the car seat and a link to find child seat fitting locations).

THE BOTTOM LINE:
Take everything you can. If you need to leave this book behind because you don't have room for it, I understand. Get another one later.

Tip #91
THE DRIVE HOME: Your First Time behind the Wheel...

THE TIP:
It just might be one of the most paranoid, surreal, mind-altering rides of your life. It will leave you on the edge of the driver's seat.

THE STORY:
The drive home was surreal, and I was paranoid. I was looking at all the other drivers, acting as if they should know

that I'm driving my child home for the first time. I'm like, "Don't you know I have a kid in the car?!" I thought braking hard would break the kid. I avoided hitting any bumps. I was driving with extreme caution. My wife and I were giddy, just cracking up. We were like, "We're driving and there's a kid in our backseat." We had no idea what we were doing. To this day, I drive differently when he's in the car. I drive slower, more cautiously, and much more deliberately, but I'm never as paranoid or hypersensitive as that day we put our son in the car for the very first time and took him home from the hospital. It was a drive more intense than drivers ed. I was on the edge of my seat and on the edge of my senses.

—Bob, son, seventeen months

✳✳✳

It's like drivers ed all over again. That moment you get everyone in the car, turn the key, and put the car in drive is the second you realize there's a baby on board. Time slows and everyone around you becomes an asshole driver.

You'll signal with precision, follow at a safe distance, stop at yellow lights, yield the right-of-way, allow cars to merge in front of you, and let people cut you off without speeding up and flipping them the bird. Lane changes are executed with extreme precision. Stop signs mean coming to a complete stop. Acceleration and braking is as smooth as butter. You will drive under the speed limit. And anyone passing, driving too fast, or looking at you the wrong way will fill you with rage—the nerve of someone to jeopardize your family's safety when all you're trying to do is drive! You've never had more precious cargo.

The drive home will be like none other. What this drive really means is:

- You are in control.
- You are at the wheel.
- You are responsible…for this child's safety, security, and well-being.

The moment you take the wheel and drive away is the moment you realize how dangerous the world can be, how much you want to protect your child from it, and how little control you have over it. The drive home isn't about operating a vehicle. It's about feeling what it means to be a father behind the wheel for the first time.

P.S. Sorry if I was ever "the other guy" driving like an asshole. I had no idea you were coming home from the hospital.

THE BOTTOM LINE:

Welcome to life behind the wheel as a new dad. It's great to have you here…

13

AFTER THE BABY IS BORN

The Fourth Trimester Begins

THE TIP:
It might not be a magical mystical experience right away.
Don't feel bad for not feeling that it is. It will be spectacular
in a few months.

THE STORY:
The coolest moment was the delivery. But the first two
months were extremely stressful and exhausting for me. I
didn't know that it's normal not to feel that magical sense.

The whole time, everyone kept telling me how great it is. Right after my son was born, it was a huge adjustment—I was in shock-and-survival mode. I was just doing whatever I could for the first two or three months. I felt an overwhelming sense of responsibility. People at work were telling me to cherish the time. I wanted to slap those people after getting two hours of sleep and feeling completely exhausted. I snapped at a few people, telling them it's really not that great. But it does get better. I can't emphasize that enough—it can take a few months until you're more confident and comfortable and in a routine. It all gets better, and it speeds up. I know that it's the last thing you want to hear for the first two or three months. I was bitter about it. Allow yourself to feel whatever you need to feel and know it will pass, and it will be better—it will be spectacular. For me, it took time. It had nothing to do with loving my kid; it was about a monumental transition, a new lifestyle, and an unprecedented sense of responsibility.

—*Josh, son, eighteen months*

***

Becoming a father is a personal experience for each new dad.

What you feel and when you feel it will vary. When it comes to the expectant father experience, we don't have much of an oral history. All we know is that life will change.

> What was interesting and took a while for me to understand was that my wife immediately had a love for and attachment to our new baby, whereas it took me a lot longer to truly love the baby in that way.
>
> —*Don, son, eight months*

> Get at least one book. Stay ahead of the timeline. Find a guru, someone who has been there before and who can answer questions, give definitions, and share recommendations.
>
> —*Dan, son, four months*

When we can get comfortable with the uncomfortable and prepare for change *before* it's time to face it, we are better equipped to alleviate stress instead of elevating it.

As a third-time father, I can tell you that different feelings will hit you at different times. But I can promise you that the overwhelming feelings will be joy and happiness. When you're feeling and experiencing new emotions, be patient, find people who can support you, and take an active role in being a dad. The information in this book will help you to be active, engaged, and find ways to be part of this experience—it's hard at first.

To help manage the changes ahead, I've listed changes to expect and a plan to help prepare for what's ahead. These are just a few suggestions. The idea is that if you know what's coming, you can do whatever fits your personality to anticipate and embrace changes as this experience unfolds.

CHANGES YOU CAN EXPECT

THE CHANGE: You'll get less attention from her.
THE ACTION PLAN: Plan how you'll be involved. Talk to her about what your roles will be. Ask her what she wants your role to be. Take a parenting class together. Pick up the book *The Happiest Baby on the Block* by Dr. Harvey Karp (more in Tip #93). Do something to be involved. Instead of watching the game or doing something on your own, take a more active role. See Tip #96 for more ideas.

THE CHANGE: She might be uncomfortable and unsure of herself in her New Mom Thong.

THE ACTION PLAN: Give her permission to be tired, hormonal, overwhelmed, emotional, irritable, and unsure of herself. Encourage her to put together a plan ahead of time—she's going to need a support system. If she doesn't have friends or family, help her find support. Connect her with other moms or professional care (see Tip #42).

THE CHANGE: You might feel financial stress.

THE ACTION PLAN: Evaluate your finances months before the baby arrives. Figure out how much things will cost and plan for the months ahead. Don't wait until you're exhausted, stressed, and overwhelmed. That's when fights happen. If you need to get a coach to help you better define your goals, then make that investment. If you have an action plan in place, you'll be focused and on track once change happens. This can mean moving, cutting expenses, or taking on extra work. See Tip #60 for more ideas.

THE CHANGE: You will be sleep-deprived.

THE ACTION PLAN: Craft a sleep strategy before you get home that will help you and your partner get more rest. Check out Tip #97 for more information.

THE CHANGE: You may be unsure of whether you're ready to be a dad.

> Your life as you know it is done. What I didn't count on, however, is how gladly and how easily I let my old life go, without a second thought. The kid makes it all worthwhile.
>
> —*Eric, son, nine months*

THE ACTION PLAN: The paternal instinct will kick in. When that switch flips on is unpredictable, but it will. Be patient and give yourself permission to take time. Talk to other guys and reach out on the Dad's Expecting Too Facebook page.

THE CHANGE: Your marriage and sex life may change.

THE ACTION PLAN: If you're worried about the relationship changing, talk to your partner about it and plan how you'll stay connected. Talk to friends or family members who have relationships you respect. Consider talking to a therapist. Once she's cleared by the doctor for sex, know that a rested happy woman is more likely to have sex. Plan for how you will help her be well rested. (See Tip #101.)

THE CHANGE: Your partner's identity will shift.

THE ACTION PLAN: This may happen because she's stopped working; because she has less time for herself, her friends, or her interests; or simply because she has this new person in her life. She simply is not the person she was before the baby. Help her come up with an action plan if she's feeling like her life is unfamiliar and overwhelming. Encourage her to talk to her friends who have been

> ## WATCH OUT FOR THE WONDER WEEKS
> There's a cool new book and website to help you understand your baby's changes during the earliest stages of development. Heads up: watch out for week 6, it's the infant's fussiest week. www.thewonderweeks.com/what-are-mental-leaps.

through this transition, and make sure you're both aware of the challenges. If you know what people trip over, you can create a new path or jump when you see it coming.

THE CHANGE: You can't hang out with friends as much.
THE ACTION PLAN: Remind yourself that this is temporary. Once you get through the first few months, things will definitely change. What might shock you is that once you have the baby, you might not want to do the things you used to do. You might not be as upset as you thought about missing a night out.

THE CHANGE: You have feelings of overwhelming responsibility.
THE ACTION PLAN: When something feels overwhelming, turn to the people who have done this before you and ask them to put things in perspective. Find out what they did right and what they did wrong. If you don't have family or friends to talk with, then find a therapist to help you deal with this. It will pass, but if your partner isn't available to talk about this and your friends aren't informed, you might need a professional.

THE CHANGE: You're stressed.
THE ACTION PLAN: Compile a list of the healthy outlets you will turn to in order to deal with the stress. Plan on going to the gym and build it into your schedule. Create a way to support your partner and still take care of yourself. Work with your partner and figure out how you can both manage it.

> No one told us that it was going to be this much fun. Most people told us how hard it would be or how little sleep we're going to get—and all of that is true, but it's just so much fun. We love having our little guy around.
>
> —*Mike, son, four months*

THE CHANGE: No one is sure how to take care of a baby at first.

THE ACTION PLAN: Research and register for a parenting class together. Pick up the book *The Happiest Baby on the Block* by Dr. Harvey Karp. Discuss this with your friends. Practice changing diapers. Taking care of a kid is a hard thing to do. Read ahead together. Make this a project you start before the baby is born. Then, when the kid arrives, you'll have a plan instead of sitting there in the middle of the night wondering what the hell to do next (I'm pointing a finger at me).

THE CHANGE: Fill in the blank at www.Dads ExpectingToo.com.

THE ACTION PLAN: Fill in the blank at www.Dads ExpectingToo.com.

THE BOTTOM LINE:

Help men (and women) understand what's coming their way by sharing your tips, stories, and experiences as they unfold (www.DadsExpectingToo.com).

THE TIP:

It's not as bad as it initially seems the first two or three days…

THE STORY:

Our daughter stayed in the room with us at the hospital. When she cried, the nurses were right there to help us. Once we lost the nurses' help, we felt overwhelmed at home. When we left the hospital, we were terrified. I remember my wife turning to me and saying, "I can't believe they're letting us leave with this little baby." When we got home, it was just the two of us. We felt all alone. We didn't think we'd need help, so we didn't ask for it. The first night was miserable. Every time we fed our daughter, she would fall asleep in our arms. Then we would put her down, and she would wake up and cry. This happened over and over again, at least fifty times, all night long. We were telling each other we couldn't do this. We didn't know if we were cut out for it. How could this be so miserable when it was all supposed to be beautiful? The second and third nights, my mom stayed with us and

I was surprised by how quickly I caught on to taking care of a baby. I'm not saying it was easy, but my son was really the first baby I had ever held. I went from thinking I was going to break him. Then I thought about the birthing process and realized after everything he's been through, I wasn't going to do too much damage to him.

—*Dan, son, two, daughter, ten months*

BACK TO SLEEP CAMPAIGN

If your baby is under twelve months old, you can help reduce the risk of SIDS (Sudden Infant Death Syndrome), suffocation, and strangulation by following these three tips:

1. Place your baby to sleep on his or her back. Babies who sleep on their backs have a much lower risk of SIDS and suffocation.
2. Remove all soft bedding from the crib. A baby can suffocate from soft bedding in a crib. Be sure to remove all pillows, quilts, comforters, and sheepskins from your crib.
3. Put your baby to sleep in a safe crib. A safe crib is the best place for your baby to sleep. Make sure your crib has no missing or broken hardware, no slats more than 2⅜ inches apart, no corner posts over ¹⁄₁₆ inch high, no cutout designs in the headboard or footboard, a firm, tight-fitting mattress, and a safety certification seal (on new cribs).

(Source: www.cpsc.gov/)

helped (she would have stayed longer, but we didn't think we'd need her), but it got better. My wife did some research and we became familiar with what our daughter wanted. It took a few nights of practice to figure it out, but we did get her to sleep. It got so much better, we decided to have a second daughter. See, it does get better.

—Thad, daughters, eleven months and three

***

They didn't give us a manual.

Neither kid came with instructions.

We were just supposed to know what to do with our newborn.

But we had no idea what the hell we were doing.

My wife was exhausted from giving birth. I was exhausted from not sleeping at the hospital. And this little person was exhausted from being evicted from the womb. We were all having our issues.

Our first three nights were spent sitting in bed with our arms crossed and our daughter nestled on our chests (accidental kangaroo care). We propped pillows under our elbows to support our arms while we half-slept. We used our knees and a pillow for additional support. The engineering ensured our daughter was safe in our arms as we slept. When we got brave, we'd place her in the co-sleeper next to the bed (a co-sleeper is like a crib that connects to the bed; the sleeping part of the name is highly deceptive). The baby never slept. The only way she would sleep was if she was resting in our arms. We knew this wasn't how it should be. But no one told us how it should be. Was this how it could be? Three nights later, we got smart—actually my wife got smart and turned to the books.

WHAT IS SIDS?

Sudden Infant Death Syndrome (SIDS) is the leading cause of death among infants aged one to twelve months and is the third leading cause overall of infant mortality in the United States. Although the overall rate of SIDS in the United States has declined by more than 50 percent since 1990, rates have declined less among non-Hispanic Black and American Indian/Alaska Native infants. African American babies die from SIDS at more than twice the rate of other babies. Preventing SIDS remains an important public health priority.

(Source: www.cdc.gov/SIDS/)

The one that saved us was *The Happiest Baby on the Block* by Dr. Harvey Karp. My wife read the important parts to me at 3:00 a.m. huddled in the bathroom (there's now a DVD too). In the book, Dr. Karp refers to the three months following birth as the fourth trimester. During the fourth trimester, the infant's calming reflex can be stimulated by applying the five S's: (1) swaddling (tight wrapping of the baby), (2) side/stomach (laying baby on her left side or stomach while awake, (3) shushing, (4) swinging, and (5) sucking.

What helped us survive:

- **Swaddling:** We kept our daughter swaddled tightly in the blanket (babies twitch and their body parts can swing around and wake them up). We got good at wrapping her up. The swaddle blankets look confining, but they were awesome.

- **Side/stomach:** Our daughter had bad reflux, so holding her on her side and stomach (while she was awake) helped calm her down.

- **Shushing:** When she cried, I would shush her again and again. Think of a silence-crazed librarian "shushing" loudly over and over again—that's how you shush.

- **Swinging:** The motion helped calm her down (swings work, our arms worked, anything that swings works).

- **Sucking:** We got her a different kind of pacifier than the one from the hospital and it made all the difference.

A second edition addition: DO NOT use a sleep positioner. While updating this book, I learned the CPSC and the U.S. Food and Drug Administration (FDA) have warned parents and caregivers to stop using sleep positioners. They pose a suffocation risk.

THE BOTTOM LINE:

Newborns don't come with user's manuals, but there are some available. Ask your doctor, friends, and family to offer suggestions. Put them in your backpack to take to the hospital. Watch *The Happiest Baby on the Block* and download it while passing time during labor (then watch the breastfeeding channel).

IMPORTANT ALERT REGARDING COSLEEPING AND FOAM MATTRESSES

The U.S. Consumer Product Safety Commission discourages parents from placing infants in adult beds. They state the risk of strangulation and suffocation. The American Academy of Pediatrics encourages room sharing, but not bed sharing. Foam mattresses pose an added danger (it's harder for an infant to move).

THE TIP:

A man needs to remind his mother that she is not the mother's mother, and the relationship between his mom and his wife will never be the same as the relationship between his wife and her mom.

THE STORY:

I knew that my mother-in-law was excited about the grandchild and helping me during my recovery, but when my ass is hurting from giving birth and I'm the one who is exhausted, I want my mommy there to take care of me, not his. We know she's there and available. We'll call when we need help. And it's his job to run interference if his mother is overbearing. (P.S. I love my mother-in-law—she's an excellent grandmother!)

—*Misti, daughter, two*

> My mother-in-law helped us out with our newborn daughter. When she left, that was the saddest I've ever been to see my mother-in-law leave.
>
> —*Thad, daughters, eleven months and three*

***

- If someone offers help, take them up on it.
- If someone offers to bring you dinner, accept it.
- If someone offers to pay for a night nurse as a gift, let them.
- If your mom or mother-in-law offers to spend a week with you, let her.

- If your mom or mother-in-law offers to spend two weeks with you, let her.
- If your partner is overwhelmed, hire help (if financially possible).
- If your partner is depressed, help her find help (see Tip #49).

Bring in the reinforcements. Take advantage of all the help you can get.

You might like the idea of spending time together as a family, but you have your entire life to be a family. Yes, there will be times when a house guest will wear out his or her welcome. There will be moments when you think it was a big mistake, but the bigger mistake is not letting people help. Even the most annoying, obnoxious, and irritating family member can be helpful. You just need to set boundaries and know that it's only temporary. Take all the help offered.

Giving birth and caring for a newborn is a different kind of work. Sleep deprivation combined with a steep learning curve can be draining at times (but worth it). Don't be a hero and tell everyone that you'll manage. Unless you manage an infant day care and are used to caring for newborns, you'll discover that newborns need constant care and attention. After the first few weeks, you'll wish you had some help. Get it sooner rather than later.

I thought we could do it on our own—and we survived, but I wasn't the one getting up

> Don't refuse help. Even if someone wants to hold the baby for a few minutes, take them up on it.
>
> —Jeff, daughter, nine months, son, five and a half

three times a night to nurse for thirty to forty-five minutes. I wasn't the one who gave birth or managed the baby's sleeping, eating, clothing, and care. She needs as much help as possible—from you, from friends, from family, from

> Shield her from constant visitors all day; only let people in who are going to help you and not tire you out by expecting you to entertain them.
>
> —*Elizabeth, daughter, seven months*

paid professionals. The rest of this chapter mentions other things you can do to help, so plan on helping. The little things will make a profound difference.

When someone asks you the question, "What can I do to help?" suggest he or she send dinner (this implies that they will not be joining you). Your partner is not going to want to cook and you're not going to want to cook. It's a luxury when meals are ready to cook or prepared for you. If someone wants to do something very special and they have a budget, ask about a night nurse. When it comes to things like cleaning the house, it might be worth hiring a service to come once every few weeks or so—this is something you can build into your budget.

Warning: Postpartum women and men can be hormonal—even more intense and powerful than during the pregnancy. The physical and emotional changes coupled with the hormonal surge can mean that your partner might say or do things that will aggravate or annoy you. You might do the same. This can be even more challenging to navigate when you're overtired and overwhelmed. The hormones will wane, but until then, allow her to be right even when she's wrong. Help her through this by allowing her to ride the hormonal highway. If at any time you think she might be suffering from postpartum depression (PPD), let her doctor know and insist she get help (see Tip #49).

THE BOTTOM LINE:

When someone asks, "Can I help?" practice saying "Yes, yes, yes!"

Tip #95
NURSING AND BOTTLE-FEEDING: Supporting Her Milky Breasts and Using a Bottle

THE TIP:

If she's breastfeeding, the onus is on her to feed your baby—no one else can do it, and that is a heavy responsibility when you're overtired.

THE STORY:

He helped me succeed because he never made negative comments; he took her downstairs when she was unsettled so I could sleep and brought her up for a feed. New babies always seem to want to be fed when your food is ready, so he often fed me while I nursed. I was also always thirsty but initially needed two hands to feed. I discovered that he is also an expert at holding a glass so I could drink without spilling down my front. Our families also took over the

> I think of breastfeeding as the biggest accomplishment of my life—bigger than college, bigger than grad school, or anything I've done in my career.
> —Stephanie, daughter, twenty-three months, twenty-five weeks pregnant

household tasks for me for the first three weeks. A man shouldn't underestimate how invaluable those small things are. I couldn't have done it without his help, and yet at the time, they seemed like such simple things to do.

—*Elizabeth, daughter, seven months*

> No one told me that I would get engorged and sore and that it would be a really awkward process for the first week or so. It's not only hard physically, it's also hard emotionally.
>
> —*Maggie, son, three months*

***

Either your baby will be on formula, breast milk, or a combination of the two.

My wife nursed for about ten months for each baby. There was never a question for her. What I soon learned is that breastfeeding can be intense and all-consuming. It was stressful to watch my wife go through it. With the baby feeding every two to three hours, she was constantly pumping, waking up, and whipping it out (her breast—and more like gently pulling it out). There were always issues that came up (clogged milk duct, thrush, engorgement). And that brings me to my next suggestion.

If your partner is breastfeeding, urge her to find a lactation consultant. They are experts who will show her how to nurse and help her should there be challenges. My wife tells everyone to get a lactation consultant. Feeding a baby

> Breastfeeding is great for some women, but not all. The most important thing is getting sleep and having a happy wife.
>
> —*Cathy, sons, four months and three and a half*

> My wife breastfed or pumped for twins for eighteen months. She was like a cow at a dairy farm. She had these pumps hooked up to herself seemingly all day long.
>
> —*Doug, daughter, three, son, three*

can be the hardest thing a new mom will do. Will she have enough milk? How do you get the best latch? What happens if her nipples crack? She needs people in her corner to help her learn how to nurse the baby and take care of herself.

As a formula-fed baby with a tobacco-scented amniotic sac (my mom was a pregnant smoker before there were warning labels), I like to use my own experience as the litmus test. Therefore, I didn't pressure her one way or the other. I do like the idea of breast milk because it can save a lot of money (formula is expensive) and it's recommended. I didn't factor in the emotional, physical, and logistical aspects of being married to a nursing woman.

Seriously, her world centered around her breasts and the baby's feeding schedule.

> Breastfeeding is not easy. It really is a commitment that both parents or partners have to support. As a dad, it can feel helpless at times. I learned to change diapers, bounce, shush, rock, and sway my daughter to help soothe her in between feedings. It made me feel connected to my daughter, and my wife appreciated the break.
>
> —*Brian, daughter, twelve months*

HOW ABOUT THOSE MILKY BREASTS...

Men can buy milk. We can't produce it.

Breasts are amazing. Besides growing large, they are smart. Nature has made it so breasts regulate their own milk production based on a baby's intake. If my daughter didn't feed for a while, my wife's breasts would become engorged and swell up to an inhuman size—think the fakest biggest breasts at a strip club in the middle of rural Nebraska (no disrespect to my wife's breasts or strip clubs in rural Nebraska). When she saw a picture of my daughter or heard my daughter's cry, her milk would "let down." Letdown is the equivalent of the dam breaking—she was ready to flow. Letdown could also mean leaking, spritzing, or spraying.

WHY BREASTFEED YOUR BABY?

1. A mother's milk has just the right amount of fat, sugar, water, and protein that is needed for a baby's growth and development. Most babies find it easier to digest breast milk than formula. Breast milk contains agents (called antibodies) that help protect infants from bacteria and viruses and help them fight off infection and disease. Human milk straight from the breast is always sterile.

2. Breastfeeding saves time and money. You do not have to purchase, measure, and mix formula, and there are no bottles to warm in the middle of the night.

3. Breastfeeding also helps a mother bond with her baby. Physical contact is important to newborns and can help them feel more secure,

WHY BREASTFEED YOUR BABY? (cont.)

warm, and comforted. Nursing uses up extra calories, making it easier to lose the pounds gained from pregnancy. It also helps the uterus get back to its original size more quickly and lessens any bleeding a woman may have after giving birth. Breastfeeding also may lower the risk of breast and ovarian cancers.

4. The U.S. Surgeon General recommends that babies be fed with breast milk only—no formula—for the first six months of life. It is better to breastfeed for six months and best to breastfeed for twelve months, or for as long as you and your baby wish. Solid foods can be introduced when the baby is six months old, while you continue to breastfeed.

(Source: www.4women.gov)

Because my wife was working, she had to do a lot of pumping. She needed to pump to keep up her milk production and to have enough milk for our daughter when she was at work. The first time, she had a pump that plugged into the wall. The second time around, pumps got fancy and wireless. This way she could pump and dance (not really dance). We were always talking about her milk production. She was like a dairy farmer. She would then take the milk and freeze it. (A side note: the first time, the freezer

SUGGESTED READING

Child of Mine: Feeding with Love and Good Sense by Ellyn Satter

broke, and she lost about forty-five ounces of breast milk. The second time, a babysitter left the freezer open, and she lost a one-week stockpile. She literally was crying over spilled thawed milk.) Oh, if possible, get a second freezer to store extra milk if your regular freezer is temperamental or you want back-up milk.

Getting a good night's sleep while nursing is tough the first couple of months. My wife was averaging about thirty minutes a feeding with each kid. Then, after feeding, she had to change the diaper and soothe the baby back to sleep. Between getting up, feeding the baby, and getting her back down, it was exhausting. This is true of all moms who get up to do feedings—not just nursing moms. The most helpful thing a man can do is to bring the baby to her in the middle of the night and put the baby back down. If he can do the feeding too, that's even more helpful.

WAYS TO SUPPORT HER AND HER BREASTS

Get an Expert Involved: She might not know how her milk-making breasts work. Suggest that she get the name of a lactation consultant before she walks into the hospital. Also, before the baby is born, see if there's a lactation consultant at the hospital. If she should have questions or a problem, turn her breasts in the direction of a consultant. Sometimes the consultation can be covered under insurance (talk to your pediatrician or caregiver).

Respect Her Choice: Don't pressure her to nurse if she's not interested. Breastfeeding takes an unwavering commitment. If she's not up for it, don't force her (although I don't think you could force her because they're her breasts).

FEEDING SUGGESTION

If you and your partner are having a hard time feeding your son or daughter, talk to a specialist as soon as possible. Many newborns can have underlying issues that can impact feeding.

Not All Women Produce Enough: Until she gives birth she won't know if she can produce milk. Even if she can produce milk, it might not be enough milk. Do not put pressure on her to nurse. If she is unable to produce enough milk, pressuring her will only make her feel like she disappointed you. She'll have a hard enough time dealing with it herself.

Bring the Baby to Her: Getting up at night and putting the baby down can take time. Even if you're working and she's working, figure out how you can help.

Bring Water to Her: She needs to stay hydrated and nourished. Get her a special mug or water bottle to help her keep up her water intake.

Buy a Breast Pump: If she's up for pumping, get a quality breast pump. There are hand breast pumps, but I imagine you would probably cramp up after an ounce or two. Electric ones are most efficient. If she can pump, then she can put some milk in a bottle and you can enjoy feeding your baby

BREASTFEEDING BOOKS

Encourage her to only read books that are recommended by a lactation consultant, doctor, or a friend who shares a similar philosophy. Some issues relating to childbirth can evoke strong emotions. Breastfeeding is one of those issues.

too. Gift idea: pimp up her pump with rhinestones for Mother's Day…

Tasting the Milk: It's kind of like sweet sugar water. I've never had a cup of breast milk or dipped Oreos in it, but I did taste it. My wife put a drop in my mouth. I gagged. There's something programmed into our heads that the milk isn't for us.

Her Enormous Milky Breasts: Milk-producing breasts can be huge, but they're better left untouched. When getting back together, consider protective eyewear and pads. Breasts spray, leak, and spritz when you least expect it.

ABOUT BOTTLE-FEEDING

Some moms will not want to breastfeed or won't produce enough milk to breastfeed. If your baby is on formula or if your nursing partner pumps, you will be lucky enough to feed the baby. Feeding a baby can be intimidating.

I'm fortunate enough to live with a feeding expert. It's not that she's an expert at feeding herself (no feeding jokes—remember, she's pregnant); my wife is a specialist in infant feeding and swallowing. She spends her time working in a rehabilitation hospital, private practice, and a

NICU helping infants and children become better eaters. Having an expert with me was so helpful when feeding and choosing the right bottle for our daughter. My wife showed me how to hold the baby, how to hold the bottle, and how the different nipples can control the flow. It's hard to know what kind of flow, nipple, and bottle will work. No one is expecting you to know, but if your partner gets frustrated, know that there are options. Feeding can be a source of stress, whether it's by bottle or nursing. If you have any

BOTTLES UP (AVOID BISPHENOL A)

When picking bottles, make sure you look at the code on the bottom and make sure they are BPA free. Plastic containers have recycle codes on the bottom. In general, plastics that are marked with recycle codes 1, 2, 3, 4, 5, and 6 are very unlikely to contain BPA. Some, but not all, plastics that are marked with recycle code 7 may be made with BPA. As of January 2009, the six major U.S. manufacturers of baby bottles and infant feeding cups have confirmed to the FDA they have not manufactured these products using BPA for the U.S. market. These manufacturers represent more than 90 percent of the U.S. market. These manufacturers produce brands that include Avent, Doctor Brown's Natural Flow, Evenflow, First Essentials, Gerber, Munchkin, Nuk, and Playtex.

issues, talk to your pediatrician and or a specialist. There are also community websites for new moms with some very active discussion boards.

If your partner is nursing and you would like to help with the feeding, ask if she can pump so you can help. If she's not comfortable pumping, bring the baby over to her to feed and then put the baby back to sleep. If the baby is formula-fed, build up your confidence early and do some feedings in the hospital when the nursing staff is available. Your style can be different than her style but still be a good style. When it comes to feeding the baby, here are the top five things you should avoid:

- Forcing a bottle in a baby's mouth when he's not taking it readily.
- Jiggling a bottle in a baby's mouth to keep her sucking.
- Trying to keep feeding a baby who is giving you signals he is all done.
- Ignoring repeated signs of trouble with feeding: frequent coughing, gagging, excessive spitting up, formula coming out the baby's nose.
- Thinking you can't feed the baby the right way—you can develop your own style; just because you do it differently doesn't mean it's wrong.

THE BOTTOM LINE:

If you pump your breasts as a gesture of support, make sure to clean the hoses thoroughly before she uses the pump again.

Tip #96
TAKE A SHIFT A WEEK: Getting Peed On, Pooped On, and Helping Out...

THE TIP:

If she's at home during the week and you're working during the week, take care of the baby at least one day on the weekend. It will give your wife time to take care of herself and find some balance—she needs it.

THE STORY:

It's hard for men to understand that taking care of a newborn can be all-consuming. It's hard to get things done. My husband would come home from work and say he's going to get a haircut, going to the cleaners, and going to exercise. And I'm like, "I've needed to do that for the last three months." Men can pick up and go whenever they want. Work obligations are work obligations, but when they're not working, it's nice when they take over. My husband didn't realize how hard it was for me to get things done until I talked to him about it. On the weekends, he'll be in charge of our son for a whole Sunday. He tells me which nights he'll be home and what's happening on the weekend in advance. Some nights, I'll go out and run my errands. So he understands. Some of my friends have told me that the only way men will understand is if you leave them alone with the kid for the entire week. Sometimes, after a long day, I want nothing to

> I've had every bodily fluid on me—poop, pee, vomit, and diarrhea. It's a rite of passage all dads experience.
>
> —*Eliot, father of two*

do with my son. I'm like, you feed him, you give him dinner, you read him stories—I just don't want anything to do with him, but I still love him.

—Tami, son, eighteen months, pregnant with number two

* * *

A babysitter is technically someone other than a mom or dad who gets paid to take care of the baby while the parents are away. Therefore, a dad is NOT a babysitter (although it might feel like it the first time). Being left alone in a room with your newborn might be a frightening thought. It's hard to know how a baby works. While intimidating to think that you are in charge for a day, there's nothing like being in charge. Do it.

- Being in charges helps you appreciate what it takes to care for a baby. Feeding the baby, changing the baby, putting the baby down for a nap, playing with the baby, and taking care of the baby all day long is a lot of work—physically and emotionally. If you have a baby who screams, it's that much more exhausting. One afternoon was all it took for me to understand—thank G-d for Elmo (he helped my daughter chill out when she lost it for forty-five minutes)!

- Being in charge will give your partner time to find

some balance. As one dad said, "It's not 24/7; it's 24/7/10,080." (The 10,080 are the minutes that make up the week.) If she's nursing, she's that much more tied to the baby. If you want her to be happy, which is essential for having a happy home, which is essential for your happiness, then she needs to find some balance. She needs time to work out, get her hair and nails done, take a nap, hang out with friends without the baby, and take a little time to renew, refresh, and get reinvigorated. Give a little, and you'll get so much back.

- Being in charge means making your own rules. You can be caring, loving, and nurturing without having to do it the way your partner does it. You might even do some things better.
- Being in charge gives you confidence. The more you can get comfortable with the uncomfortable, the better equipped you'll be to handle future situations. Like when your daughter brings home a boy in seventeen years. (Scream, it's okay!)
- Being in charge helps you get messy. If you're lucky, while you're taking care of your kid, he or she might cry, spit up, vomit, pee, poop, or have diarrhea on you. And yes, I've actually caught vomit in my hands without spilling. I made it to the sink without any dripping (a proud moment).

> I never minded changing my son's diaper. With my daughter, I'm afraid of hurting her and you don't know how it all works—it can be a little intimidating.
>
> —*Mark, son, two and a half, daughter, ten months*

THE BOTTOM LINE:

Getting peed, pooped, vomited, and thrown up on is a rite of passage.

Tip #97
SLEEPING AND NOT SLEEPING: Crafting a Sleep Strategy before Getting Sleepy

THE TIP:

A man should realize that mom needs time to get healthy and heal; otherwise recovery is going to be a lot longer.

THE STORY:

Our first daughter was colicky and cried for hours on end. It was very overwhelming for us. She wouldn't stop crying. She was high-maintenance since day one and still is. We had a hard time settling whose turn it was to hold her and who gets out of the house. We ended up taking turns at night when it came to sleeping. I would get the first half of the night to sleep and he would get the second half of the night. At least we would each get about five straight hours. Our second two were angels because we weren't so tense. He was very helpful with all three and it made it manageable.

—Joann, daughters, two (twins) and four

Let's start with the basics:

- A newborn will sleep roughly sixteen hours a day.
- Sleep will be in two- to four-hour stretches at a time.
- Figure that a feeding takes thirty to forty-five minutes.
- For every eight hours of uninterrupted sleep you get, she may sleep for a total of five to six interrupted hours (this is factoring in three feedings and changing and

soothing the baby back to sleep after each feeding).

All this sleeping will screw up your schedule. Newborns will nap more than a kid home from college during winter break. They have about sixty minutes of awake time and then they sleep. It's a little ridiculous.

SUGGESTED SLEEP MUSIC

Lullaby by Justin Roberts. This soothing album by Grammy-nominated Justin Roberts features beautiful arrangements that put you and your baby in dreamland. Visit www.JustinRoberts.com or download online.

I fought this early on, and it caused a lot of problems. Having sixty minutes of awake time meant that we didn't have a lot of time to go out and do things. Some moms don't mind if a baby sleeps in the car seat, but other moms want the baby home in the crib (it all depends on what sleep training method you follow—yes, there are training methods). My wife was 100 percent right, but I never took the time to read the sleep training books. Instead, I just resisted the method. As a result, I turned my wife into the bad guy when she would insist on putting our daughter down for nap time. I still feel bad that I put her in that position.

Do yourself a favor and either play an active role in researching methods with her or respect her way of running the show. And then, when you're out with grandparents and they want to push the baby to stay up a little later, instead of letting her take the heat, explain that loving their grandchild should mean wanting their grandchild to get a good night's sleep and not be overtired and cranky the next morning.

You would think, with the baby sleeping so much, you would get a lot of sleep, but newborns are unpredictable sleepers. A colicky baby or a newborn with excessive reflux can cry for hours and hours at a time (those are the wakeful hours). You won't know what kind of baby you have until you meet him or her, but in the meantime you can prepare for what's ahead.

> The biggest challenge was SLEEP—for us and the baby. I was so naive. I honestly thought that the baby would only wake up once a night because I only woke up once a night during my pregnancy.
>
> —*Megan, daughter, eleven months*

Talk to a hundred guys and ask them if they had a sleep strategy when they came home, and they'll tell you that they were lucky to remember the car seat. Devising a sleep strategy is not something most of us think about ahead of time—mainly because no one tells us we should.

All anyone tells us is how tired we will be when the baby gets here. They don't tell us how to avoid being tired. You are not going to get as much sleep as you got before the baby arrived, but you can get more sleep than the guys complaining about it if you do some planning. Without a plan, you can plan on being sleep-deprived.

Sleep is hard to come by the first few months (it will get better). But there is sleep to be had. There is a way to make this work, or at least pretend that it can work.

> I was so sleep-deprived I drove away after pumping gas with the nozzle still in the gas tank of my car.
>
> —*Gary, sons, six months and three*

Until you know if you have a good sleeper, it's hard to know if you'll get some good sleeping in. Before you leave the hospital (or wherever you have this baby), develop a sleep strategy. Talk to friends, family, your doctor, or midwife.

Here are some strategies that may help you find some sleep:

- Take as much time as possible during the first couple of weeks and help her to heal so she can get her strength back.
- You need to figure out how the baby works so that you can get comfortable helping her out during the first week or two.
- Whoever is working gets to sleep during the week. Whoever is working as the primary caregiver does weeknight feedings. If the working partner can help during weeknights and still be functional, even better.
- On the weekends, whoever was working does the night-time feedings. If that's not possible because your partner is nursing, this means helping her by bringing the baby to her (so she can get more sleep), and it means giving her time to nap during the weekend.
- The rule: caregivers nap when the baby is napping (as long as you're not out shopping—do not nap in department stores).
- Sleep in shifts or sleep in separate rooms. There's no

reason for two people to be exhausted. Over the weekend, it will be her turn to sleep in (assuming she's on maternity leave).

- Once one of you returns to work, if sleep is an issue, consider getting a night nurse once a week for a few weeks. If two sets of grandparents are available, have one set help out the first week and the other help the second week. Then rotate them back through until you can handle it on your own.
- Get some sleep books and read them. Swaddling, soothing, and kangaroo care are a few strategies that can help. Gather techniques and ideas from friends, family, and the pros so you're ready before you need it.
- Read the sleeping techniques in Tip #93 and *The Happiest Baby on the Block*—that book saved our lives.
- Talk to your pediatrician or family doctor. Sometimes kids who can't sleep could be having other issues. They might be able to offer you some suggestions that will make this transition easier.

THE BOTTOM LINE:
Don't stay up too late creating your sleep strategy.

Tip #98
WORKING AT HOME: Setting Up a Conference Call during Nap Time

THE TIP:
It might not work out according to the plan. It may take time to figure it out.

THE STORY:

My wife works full time and I work from a home office half the year. The plan was for her to work from home on Fridays and take care of him while getting work done. The expectation was that I would also help watch the baby while trying to get work done. It turned out that neither one of us could get anything done. Between feeding him and playing with him, it was impossible. One Friday, she was out running some errands while I was working at home. I had a conference call scheduled during his nap time. Well, that day he woke up early from his morning nap hungry and crying. I also needed to take this call. The only way I could keep him quiet was to feed him during the conference call. I was staring at him in the eyes begging him not to cry. I'm sure the people on the call heard some feeding baby noises, but there wasn't anything else I could do. After this incident, I pretty much told my wife that I can't take care of him and work. She couldn't get anything done either and respected it. We made adjustments. Now, on Fridays, we drop off our son at her parents' house after playing and eating breakfast in the morning. It took a while to figure out how to make it work.

—*Irl, son, twenty-two months, twenty-eight weeks pregnant*

✳✳✳

If you're not a full-time dad, you'll be going back to work. For me, work meant going upstairs to my office. Unless you run a daycare center, working at home with a baby in the house makes it hard to get work done. I tried. I found home to be the black hole of cuteness and things "to do."

Babies are too cute to avoid. There's always something happening. A smile, a crawl, or a step. And my wife always had something for me to get done. After my second kid was born, I was forced out of the house. It was the best thing that could have happened. I never realized how much being at home made it hard to work. As a pro, here are some suggestions to work at home and stay in business.

> She comes home with the groceries, and I help put away the groceries. Then I play with my son. And before I know it, I've been away from work for three hours.
>
> —Matt, sons, one month and two and a half

SET BOUNDARIES

There will be times you want to take a break and play with your newborn. Before you know it, you'll be changing a diaper, soothing a crying baby, preparing a bottle, putting together a new toy, and jumping around like an idiot. Then the phone will ring and you'll remember that you're supposed to be at work. When you get back to work, you'll realize it's time to stop working because it's the end of the day.

The next problem is that your partner might distract you (even if she's not trying to). Having you around means that you're, well, around. And being accessible means that it's easy to call out to you when a cute thing happens, or when she needs more diapers, or when you need to bring up clothes, make a bottle, or help during a crisis. Being at home with a sick kid…well, forget it—not getting called into a vomit or explosive poop episode is impossible. Setting boundaries can be a challenge.

DISCUSS ERRANDS AND APPOINTMENTS

Talk about what's going on during the week on Sunday night. Also talk about what your partner expects you to do or not do. If your partner is on maternity leave, she might want to run an errand, get her hair cut, or have lunch with a friend. She might schedule a service call or some kind of delivery. She might want to run out to the gym for an hour. This means you need to be home (and not working). Discuss this with her ahead of time and work out a plan. Otherwise, when she has a doctor's appointment, you will find yourself putting the baby down for a nap at the same time you have a conference call planned.

GET OUT OF THE HOUSE

Get used to getting out of the house. Set some dedicated time to not be home working. Go to a coffee shop or a restaurant with Wi-Fi. These days, you can pretty much take your computer and go online almost anywhere.

STRUCTURE THE DAY

Have breakfast together, have lunch together, and set a quitting time. It might vary, but if your partner knows that you have structure, she can check with you first when she needs you to do something during the day, or she can save it for later. The structure is as much for you as it is for those sharing the house and space with you.

FORWARD A BIZ CALL TO CELL

The secret is to work at home and never have anyone know that you're working at home. If you're on the phone with a client, the baby screaming and the dog barking won't do anything to help you close the deal—unless you're supposed to be working at a kennel or daycare facility. Make sure you use your cell phone as your primary line or have your business line forward to your cell phone during noisy times. This way, you can always leave the room if someone or something gets too noisy.

GET AN OFFICE

I know you don't want to take on the expense of an office after taking on the expense of a baby, but sometimes being home can reduce productivity to the point that the expense of moving out becomes an investment to increase productivity. Keep the thought at the back of your mind. You might be increasing expenses, but you'll ultimately increase revenue.

THE BOTTOM LINE:

You can have breakfast, lunch, and dinner with your new family and still be able to pay for breakfast, lunch, and dinner working from home.

Tip #99
THE FULL-TIME DAD—aka the Do-It-All Dad

THE TIP:

Your wife and friends will be jealous.

THE STORY:

I decided to stay at home because my wife now makes about seven times what I was making and she travels a lot for work. I hated my job and waited until they fired me (to get unemployment), which was about a month before the second baby was born. My responsibilities are to the kids and the house (and dog). I don't have clients who need things. My older son and I can play sports and video games together. My wife is jealous, because she wanted to be the stay-at-home mom. I told her to quit; we'd move to a smaller house and stop vacations, dinners, etc. She'd rather have the money. My friends are jealous. I call them during the day to ask if they can go to an early afternoon baseball game or to the race track, and they are busy at work (I have a sitter come in once a week). When the baby sleeps, then I can read, play on the computer, or go to sleep. I went to the first PTA meeting of the year. Out of forty-three people, I was the only man. On school field trips, I'm the only dad. Most moms think it's great (at least that's what they tell me) that I stay home with the kids. All that matters is what my wife thinks. The one thing they don't understand is that when the baby is not sleeping, I'm not sleeping. This week, the kids have been sick, and I've been suffering from major sleep deprivation. I must admit, I do enjoy that some of my male friends are jealous.

—Jeff, daughter, seven months, son, five

✳✳✳

Becoming a full-time dad might have never even crossed your mind until reading this. You might be thinking you'd love to do this, but you don't want to "stay at home." However stay-at-home dads are allowed to go out and do a lot of things. They can go shopping, go to the park, and go to sporting events in the afternoon (if you get a sitter).

Given that 33 percent of the workforce is working at home, a lot of full-time workers are part-time stay-at-home dads and don't even know it. I don't even think they realize it. Their employers don't realize it either, but fathers' roles are constantly shifting. With the Internet, cell phones, and laptops, you can work during nap times, while waiting in the car during carpools, or after bed-time. For couples who work different shifts (mom works days and dad works nights), the father is playing a larger role. Then there are dads who are the primary caregivers

A FULL-TIME DAD SEES THE WORLD

My wife and I decided that I would be a full-time dad. I say I love my job and there isn't anything else I would rather be doing. My kids will only be this young once and I do not want to miss it. I love my wife and think we have a perfect situation, with her playing to her strengths and me to mine. Without her success and dedication, our family would not be able to enjoy all the things we do. We are all very lucky and happy together. Here are the more common reactions you'll get when someone discovers you're a full-time dad:

From Dads:

1. A quick change of conversation.
2. "Man, that must be awesome. I wish I could do that. I would play golf and go to the gym, catch up on the movies I haven't seen." When I reply, "Who would watch your kids during all these activities?" I am greeted with silence and then the realization that what I do might be a job after all.
3. There have been times when I have hung out with my kids and their friends so much that when we are at a park and the kids say hi to me, the dads wonder who is this guy their kids all know.

A FULL-TIME DAD SEES THE WORLD (cont.)

From Moms:

1. "That is so wonderful, I wish my husband could do that, but he's useless."
2. Some are mistrustful and think I am some sort of deviant.
3. Most are cool with it, and eventually accept me into their circle of friends.

From Nannies:

1. Friendly or feeling threatened that if this trend catches on, the stay-at-home dads might put the nannies out of business.

My Wife:

1. She loves the situation and refers to her time alone with the kids as "babysitting."
2. She does wonder why all the moms of the kids our children are friends with are attractive. I say, "I never noticed."

—Jon, son, nine, daughter, seven

over the weekend. The reality is that the line between the working-outside-the-home dad and the stay-at-home dad has been so blurred that it's time for a new expression. I just don't think the term stay-at-home dad is appropriate anymore. How about a do-it-all dad? That seems much more appropriate.

Given the significant role we play in the pregnancy experience, it's not surprising that more men are sticking around and wanting to stick around. Do-it-all dads (formerly known as stay-at-home dads) can find support groups, conventions, forums, and organizations where they can share information with other dads. Whether the choice is made for financial or personal reasons, I've never met a guy who has said it sucked. I'm sure there are some out there (it's nice to meet you all) who don't like it, but it's not a bad life. As technology makes us more independent and mobile, I wouldn't be surprised to see fathers working shorter weeks or perhaps shifting their work hours to after bedtime and spending more time with their kids. There's no shame in being actively involved and engaged in your child's life. I think it's cool.

THE BOTTOM LINE:

Being a full-time dad lasts eighteen years. Then you have the rest of your life to work in an office.

Tip #100
WORKING ON THE ROAD: Being There When You're Not Really There...

THE TIP:

When on the road, take advantage of technology to help you stay connected.

THE STORY:

I'm probably on the road over a hundred days a year. One of the things we've been doing to help deal with it is video conferencing. A few months after the baby was born, we got two Mac laptops. It's made a huge difference. I kind of know the baby's nap schedule, so if it's before 9:26 a.m. Nashville time, I can tell my wife I'm online. She'll turn on the computer, and then I'll play with my daughter. We'll wave to each other and play peekaboo. I'll bounce from bed to bed making her giggle. It's a strange way of doing it, but I get to play with my baby. When I log off, I'm all alone in my hotel room, and that's kind of weird. We use technology to make it work with me being on the road. It also helps me to stay more connected with my wife. There will be times when I can chat with her for an hour and a half. We'll talk about stuff that we need to figure out—finances, the baby, her new business, and other issues. I can be supportive of her. Of course, it's no substitute for being a husband or father who is home all the time, but it's been great to interact this way when I'm away.

—*Jason, daughter, twelve months*

***

I love technology. I devour it. I've had dinner with my kids while working out on an elliptical machine. I've read stories to them while they're at home and I'm in some god-forsaken city in the middle of nowhere. I've watched class recitals, listened to their problems, and heard about their days while I look into their eyes. We've also gone on roller coasters, dived underwater, and traveled to the moon together (thanks, Apple). I

THINGS TO DO TO HELP WHEN YOU TRAVEL

- Make meals and freeze them.
- Video chat and give her a break.
- Suggest she get a sitter a couple of hours a day.
- Videotape messages for the baby.

can be present in my kids' lives without being in the same zip code and I'm grateful for this.

Being on the road doesn't mean being away. FaceTime, Skype, and Google+ make it easy to have dinner, tell stories, and tuck kids in at night. It's the closest thing to being there without physically being there. Plus, you get a good night's sleep. Because of advances in technology, working on the road doesn't mean being as far away.

But not being there means that you can't help out. You can't support her during a 3:00 a.m. feeding, you can't soothe the baby when she's crying for three hours, and you can't be there to watch the baby while your partner runs out for a second.

If you have to travel, make sure she has support. When you're away, she's not going to have a break. In addition to being there online and on the phone for her, it's important that she has someone else available at home when you're away for long periods

> Those years of staying at home are precious to me and a privilege that most men don't get.
> —*David, father of two*

of time. This could mean encouraging her to have a sitter a couple times a week so she can get things done. Ask your family and friends to check in with her and drop by when you're not around. If you don't know a lot of people, make an effort through work friends to connect her with people with whom she has something in common. If you don't live near family, it could mean thinking about a possible move so that she can find support while you're gone. Also, encourage her to reach out and see if there are new mom groups, playgroups, or groups where she can meet people with whom she shares common interests.

When you get home from being on the road, as exhausted as you might be, recognize that she's going to need some help. Offer to take the baby for the day or a few hours and encourage her to do whatever she wants to do so she can have time for herself. It's not that she can't take care of the baby; it's just that being a mom 24/7 and not being able to have balance can leave her feeling like she's going out of her mind. I do a lot of speaking events and traveling. I love my job, but I don't love being away from the people whom I love the most in life. I was fortunate enough to meet a woman whose dad had been on the road her entire life. I asked her the question "Is it hard having a dad who travels so much?" She replies, "People ask me that question a lot. I have to tell you, it's the best. I have friends who have dads who work forty hours a week at home and they don't ever talk. When my dad is home, he's really home. We do things. We talk. I wouldn't trade that for anything." I thanked her. She had no idea how much that meant to me.

THE BOTTOM LINE:
No matter how many miles away, dads can be closer to home than ever before.

Tip #101
HAVING SEX AGAIN (WITH HER): The Sexual Hibernation Is Over

THE TIP:
Typically, postbaby moms are very happy to wait past six weeks. Some women schedule their appointment at seven weeks to give them extra time.

THE STORY:
I wasn't looking forward to having sex again following the birth, physically or emotionally. It was intimidating and the furthest thing from my mind. The first time we had sex it was like sandpaper; it was dry and it hurt. It took probably a good three or four months for it to not hurt. I wanted to be close to my husband and get past the pain, but for a while kind of dreaded the experience. All my estrogen was going toward breastfeeding and not sex. When I stopped nursing, the sexual desire came back to me and I was finally interested in sex again. I found my husband attractive again. I remember I actually felt a crush on my trainer one week and I was like "MEN, MEN—yay, my

hormones are back." Be gentle, be patient, don't pester her, and go slow; it can be a traumatic experience.

—*Courtney, sons, six weeks, twenty-nine months*

✻✻✻

Soon it will be time for the six-week checkup—also known as the "sex week checkup."

The six-week checkup is generally when the doctor will check her out and give her the "all clear" or the "not clear" for you to get back to making another baby. Before you take a running start from across the bedroom, know that the doctor doesn't control her vagina. Even if she gets the all clear, she might not be ready for you yet. It might be weeks or even months.

Whatever you do, don't take it personally. I know, it's easy to think that you've been patient and you deserve this, but in her eyes, she deserves to sleep and relax. At six weeks, she might be exhausted, overwhelmed, and stressed out. She might feel uncomfortable with her body. She might be emotionally exhausted. She might be self-conscious of how it will feel. She could be worried about pain if she had tearing, dryness, an episiotomy, or a difficult labor.

Start slow, keep your expectations to a minimum, and see where that takes you (turn to Tip #57). Be patient and don't pressure her. It could be weeks or months until she's up for the

> If your wife is a stay-at-home mom, it will be a while before she is affectionate again. Give her a little alone time and she may be more responsive to your touch.
>
> —*Misti, daughter, two*

sexual energy you've been building up for the past few months. The better rested, more comfortable, and more relaxed she feels, the better your chances of reawakening your sexual beast from its deep hibernation. If she's slow to get back to sex, it's normal.

If you can't get past the image of her BV burned into your mind, focus on the SV (see p. 43). It might take a few weeks, but it will all come back to you.

Once she's ready to resume activity, it's a good idea to have lubrication on hand, especially if she's breastfeeding. Women who are breastfeeding may have dryness. Go slowly and listen to her closely. Let her set the pace. She might feel some discomfort. She might be sensitive. Even if she doesn't feel discomfort, the idea of sex after delivering vaginally can be an emotional hurdle.

If you find that you've gone a long period of time and she's still not comfortable, consider talking to a couples' therapist together. Find someone who specializes in postpartum intimacy issues and work through it together.

Once your sex life starts up again, know that she can get pregnant. There's a misconception that women who breastfeed can't get pregnant. NOT TRUE. Women who are breastfeeding can get pregnant. Unless you want to be flipping back to page one in a few weeks, you need to use some kind of birth control.

THE BOTTOM LINE:

The first time back isn't sex—it's called making love. Tell her that and see if she gets in the mood...

THE TIP:

We are a family, but we will always be a couple.

THE STORY:

I've seen how it works with empty nesters. Once the kids have gone, the focus turns back to each other, and unfortunately, when that focus turns back, you may find that you don't have a lot in common, which leads to problems. We try to combat this by having a date night—we go to a movie, go to dinner, and just get away. It's hard to do because I work more hours a week than I can even tell you. She works in finance, so tax season is crazy for her. And we have two kids. We're lucky we have family close by, and I have students I can trust. The whole experience of being part of the labor and delivery and having two kids has shown me a different side of my wife that makes us even closer. Being a couple is something that we always work on because we know it's something we always want to work.

—Craig, sons, seven months and two and a half

Once upon a time, you went on a date. One thing led to another and you got her pregnant (or if you're a same-sex couple, you decided to

> Laugh. If you can't laugh your way through it, you are doomed.
> *—Doug, daughter, three, son, three*

have a baby). The kid was born. And your lives were changed forever.

Most couples forget to go on dates. Spending quality time together gets lost somewhere in the middle of caring for the baby, sleeping, eating, feeding, showering, pumping (if nursing), grocery shopping, managing the house, working, working out, working out the baby's sleep schedule (with you), and adjusting to the role of being a mom or dad.

DON'T TALK ABOUT IT, DO IT

A lot of new moms do not like the idea of being away from their baby. Just the thought will send them into a panic. Arrange a sitter and plan the date. Make it for a couple of hours and within a few minutes of home. Tell her you're going on a date and then go…

Weekends are no longer about deciding which restaurant to go to, what movie to see, or the best live music to hear—they're about catching up on sleep and taking care of the bare essentials. While her world is a whirlwind, you've got a long list of issues running through your mind (see Tip #92). Everyone is consumed with other things.

And it's not like you're as physically connected during the first couple of months following the birth. There isn't any sex happening the first month. Even if she wanted to have sex, there's a pretty good chance it's too soon to do it. If your partner is the social planner, she might be too preoccupied to make plans for a romantic evening out. This means you need to make the date. And with no prospect of getting lucky, the date is solely about spending time together.

For possibly the first time in your relationship, being a

couple means making an effort and planning ahead. This idea of having to plan and make an effort is a dramatic shift that most couples don't anticipate. Before you were parents, you could do whatever you wanted whenever you wanted. Spontaneity was part of the plan. Once you have a child, spending time together as a couple isn't as automatic because there's always someone else to consider. Yes, you can take newborns to dinner or lunch and they might sleep, but it's not the same. A date is the two of you. This takes effort and deliberate planning. That's not a bad thing—it's part of being in a relationship. Just know that making time to spend together takes effort.

So make the effort.

Do whatever you can to plan a date. Have a family member watch the baby or get a sitter for a couple of hours. If she's nursing and has to pump, make it a short date. A date during the first few months following the birth isn't necessarily dinner and a movie. It can be anything as long as you're doing it together.

Some date ideas include:

- Running errands together (it makes it not a chore)
- Taking a walk
- Scheduling a couple's massage
- Hanging out at a bookstore together
- Sharing a quiet cup of coffee
- Having dessert at your favorite restaurant
- Grabbing a fast (or slow) lunch
- Having a fast (or slow) dinner
- Shopping for shoes with her (if she's not up for clothing shopping)

Since the center of attention is the baby, it's easy to forget to be a couple. It takes effort to stay connected. A little effort will mean so much to her. She might resist a little, but once she breaks free, she'll love you for it.

THE BOTTOM LINE:
If you want to spend the rest of your life together, plan on dating for the rest of your life.

Tip #103
Your Tip and Story Go Here

Welcome to the end of this book and the beginning of your experience.

As you continue on your journey, share tips and stories that will help others anticipate, embrace, and manage the changes to come. The goal is to create the most valuable resource to help men (and their partners) navigate the expectant father process. Please visit www.DadsExpectingToo .com to share your tips and stories. From your most memorable accidental asshole moment to the things you wish I had included in the book, please send it my way for consideration in future editions of this book.

Thank you!
Harlan Cohen

Looking for more great features to help you prep for your new arrival? Get the *Dad's Expecting Too* week-by-week pregnancy tracker, designed for dads and their partners, along with weekly updates about baby, your partner, and you at DadsExpectingToo.com.

✳✳✳

To get the latest news, info, facts, and stats for new and expecting parents, follow @DadsExpecting on Twitter and check out the Dad's Expecting Facebook Page at www.Facebook.com /DadsExpecting.

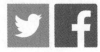

RESOURCES

WEBSITES WORTH CHECKING OUT

When doing searches for medical information, make sure you are getting information from a trusted source. My criteria of a trusted source is one that has been medically reviewed and contains current information.

FACEBOOK GROUPS

Facebook is an amazing resource. It can be helpful for you or your partner. If you're not on Facebook, sign up for an account and investigate key groups. You will be surprised how easy it is to connect with people who are dealing with similar issues. This is particularly valuable for your partner. Please join the Dad's Expecting Too Facebook Fan group, and I will include a list of valuable resources, tips, and information.

GENERAL INFORMATION

Medline Plus: www.nlm.nih.gov/medlineplus/
Centers for Disease Control: www.cdc.gov
National Institutes of Health: www.nih.gov
American Academy of Pediatrics: www.aap.org
Kids Health: www.kidshealth.org
The National Women's Health Information Center:
    www.4women.gov/pregnancy/
WebMD: www.webmd.com
The Mayo Clinic: www.mayoclinic.com
The Baby Center: www.babycenter.com
The Bump: www.thebump.com
March of Dimes: www.marchofdimes.com
About.com: pregnancy.about.com
iVillage.com: www.iVillage.com
Dad's Expecting Too: www.DadsExpectingToo.com

BIRTH LOCATION AND TEAM

Birthing Centers—American Association of Childbearing
    Centers: www.birthcenters.org
Homebirth—American College of Nurse-Midwives:
    www.midwife.org
American Academy of Family Physicians: www.aafp.org
American College of Obstetricians & Gynecologists:
    www.acog.org
Doulas of North America: www.dona.org
SheKnows Pregnancy and Baby:
    www.pregnancyandbaby.com
Midwives Alliance of North America: www.mana.org
American College of Nurse-Midwives: www.midwife.org
North American Registry of Midwives: www.narm.org

BREASTFEEDING/NURSING
LaLeche League International: www.lalecheleague.org
American Academy of Pediatrics:
   www.healthychildren.org/English/ages-stages/baby
   /breastfeeding/Pages/default.aspx
Best For Babes Foundation: www.bestforbabes.org
International Lactation Consultants Association:
   www.ilca.org

CAR SEAT SAFETY
National Highway Traffic Safety Administration:
   www.nhtsa.gov/Safety/CPS
U.S. Department of Transportation: www.safercar.gov

CHILDBIRTH EDUCATION
Your local hospital's website
American Academy of Husband-Coached Childbirth:
   www.bradleybirth.com
Lamaze International: www.lamaze.org
American Red Cross (Infant CPR/Choking):
   www.redcross.org
CPR:
   www.depts.washington.edu/learncpr/infantcpr.html

COMPLICATIONS
CDC/Centers for Disease Control and Prevention:
   www.cdc.gov (search keywords)
Diabetes/American Diabetes Association:
   www.diabetes.org
Gestational Hypertension/Preeclampsia Foundation:
   www.preeclampsia.org

Hepatitis B/Hepatitis B foundation: www.hepb.org
Preterm Labor/March of Dimes:
   www.marchofdimes.com
See general info resources above

CORD BLOOD STORAGE
Public—National Marrow Donor Program:
   http://bethematch.org
Parent's Guide to Cord Blood Foundation:
   www.parentsguidecordblood.org

DEPRESSION
Mental Health America: www.mentalhealthamerica.net
National Institutes of Mental Health:
   www.nimh.nih.gov
Postpartum Support International: www.postpartum.net

FOOD SAFETY
Federal Department of Agriculture (FDA):
   www.fda.gov/food/resourcesforyou/healtheducators
   /ucm081785.htm
FDA (for women and childcare providers):
   www.foodsafety.gov/poisoning/risk/pregnant/

HEALTH INSURANCE
Federal government website managed by the U.S.
   Centers for Medicare & Medicaid Services:
   www.healthcare.gov/

MATERNITY CLOTHES
Gap Maternity: www.gap.com

Old Navy Maternity: www.oldnavy.com
Ann Taylor Loft Maternity:
   www.anntaylorloft.com/maternity
Mimi Maternity: www.mimimaternity.com
Motherhood Maternity: www.motherhood.com
A Pea in the Pod: www.apeainthepod.com
Belly Dance Maternity: www.bellydancematernity.com/

PARENTING HELP
The Happiest Baby on the Block:
   www.thehappiestbaby.com

PATERNITY LEAVE
Department of Labor:
   www.dol.gov/dol/topic/benefits-leave/fmla.htm
National Partnership for Women & Families:
   www.nationalpartnership.org
Families & Work Institute: www.familiesandwork.org

PREGNANCY LOSS
March of Dimes: www.marchofdimes.com

PRENATAL AND GENETIC TESTING
Chicago Center for Jewish Genetic Disorders:
   www.jewishgenetics.org
Cystic Fibrosis Foundation: www.cff.org
March of Dimes: www.marchofdimes.com
National Library of Medicine's Genetic Reference site:
   http://ghr.nlm.nih.gov
National Down Syndrome Society: www.ndss.org
National Tay-Sachs and Allied Diseases: www.ntsad.org

Sickle Cell Disease Association of America:
www.sicklecelldisease.org
National Newborn Screening and Genetics Resource
Center (NNSGRC): http://genes-r-us.uthscsa.edu

SHOPPING FOR BABY

Baby Bargains: www.babybargains.com

RECOMMENDED READING:

Solve Your Child's Sleep Problems: New, Revised, and Expanded Edition—by Richard Ferber, M.D.

Baby Bargains, 7th Edition: Secrets to Saving 20% to 50% on Baby Furniture, Gear, Clothes, Toys, Maternity Wear, and Much More!—by Denise and Alan Fields

The Happiest Baby on the Block: The New Way to Calm Crying and Help Your Newborn Baby Sleep Longer—by Harvey Karp, M.D.

Mayo Clinic Guide to a Healthy Pregnancy—by Mayo Clinic

Baby 411: Clear Answers & Smart Advice For Your Baby's First Year—by Denise Fields and Ari Brown, M.D.

Pregnancy Blues: What Every Woman Needs to Know about Depression During Pregnancy—by Shaila Kulkarni Misri, M.D.

The No-Cry Sleep Solution: Gentle Ways to Help Your Baby Sleep Through the Night—by Elizabeth Pantley

Child of Mine: Feeding with Love and Good Sense— by Ellyn Satter

The Vaccine Book: Making the Right Decision for Your Child—by Robert Sears, M.D.

Healthy Sleep Habits, Happy Child—by Marc Weissbluth, M.D.

The Wonder Weeks: How to Stimulate Your Baby's Mental Development and Help Him Turn His 10 Predictable, Great, Fussy Phases into Magical Leaps Forward—by Hetty van de Rijt, Frans Plooij

The Blessing of a Skinned Knee: Using Jewish Teachings to Raise Self-Reliant Children—by Wendy Mogel, Ph.D.

Protecting the Gift: Keeping Children and Teenagers Safe (and Parents Sane)—by Gavin de Becker

EXPECTANT DAD'S DICTIONARY

As an expectant father, you'll come across words and expressions that aren't all that familiar to you. To help, we've indexed all the keywords (see index) and I've written a song you can sing during the ride to the hospital (or birthing facility). This is sung to the tune of "Supercalifragilisticexpialidocious" (from *Mary Poppins*). If you would like to record this and send it to me, I will share it with the world. ☺

Expectantfathersdosomuchbutnoonethinksaboutus
(sung to the tune of "Supercalifragilisticexpialidocious")

The layette's newborn clothing, epidurals numb her pain.
A registered nurse midwife's like a doctor—not the same.
Doulas do the coaching and Lamaze class helps her breathe.
Episiotomies will make the perineum bleed.

That perineum's skin between her buttocks and her crotch,
If baby's too big, they will cut and she will say, "Ouch."
But if she's drugged and numbed, an epidural in her spine,
The pain will be more tolerable, and ohhh she'll feel so fine.

Expectantfathersdosomuchbutnoonethinksaboutus...
If we say it loud enough, they'll curse us out and cuss us.
Expectantfathersdosomuchbutnoonethinksaboutus...
If we say it loud enough, they'll curse us out and cuss us.

The cervix, that's the opening to her uterus.
When it dilates 10 centimeters—almost time to push.
But first it must efface, that's when the cervix gets sooooo thin.
AND then it's time for pushing, let the screaming now begin.

Three stages of labor and delivery, that's what she will go through.
Stage one: labor and transition, pushing, that's number two.
Cut the cord and say hello—but wait there's still stage three.
The placenta and the afterbirth comes,
then you'll shout with glee.

Choose a water birth or home birth (please cover up the floor).
A natural birth means that she'll leave pain killers at the door.
Medically assisted births can leave her numb below the waist.
A C-section means the baby will come from a different place.

Expectantfathersdosomuchbutnoonethinksaboutus…
If we say it loud enough, they'll curse us out and cuss us.
Expectantfathersdosomuchbutnoonethinksaboutus…
If we say it loud enough, they'll curse us out and cuss us.

Big engorged breasts spritz and spray, leaking happens too.
Clogged milk ducts can cause mastitis, an infection, yep, it's true.
Stitches, bleeding, hemorrhoids from delivery they can linger.
When applying hemorrhoid cream and
witch hazel gladly lend a finger.

No sex, sleep deprivation, colicky baby crying on your lap.
It seems so rough, but it's not tough, that's if you take a nap.
But when you look in baby's eyes, you'll see what that love can do.
Just wait a year and then you'll be expecting number two!

HARLAN CAN SPEAK AT YOUR EVENT

Harlan has been entertaining and informing audiences with his keynotes, events, and workshops. Harlan can customize a program to fit the needs of your group or organization at conferences, conventions, and seminars.

Topics Harlan addresses:

GENERAL AUDIENCES:

- **Dad's Expecting Too!:** An Expectant Couple's Guide to The Expectant Parent Experience
- **Dad's Expecting Too! For Moms:** What Every Mom-to-Be Needs to Know about Her Man

FOR CAREGIVERS:

- **Dad's Expecting Too!:** What Expectant Fathers Want, Expect, and Need from Caregivers

ADDITIONAL KEYNOTES AND PROGRAMS:

Based on Harlan's bestselling book (*The Naked Roommate*) and syndicated advice column (Help Me, Harlan!).

- **Training for the Sport of Taking Risks:** How to Always Win, Regardless of the Score
- **Getting Naked:** Five Steps to Finding The Love of Your Life (While Fully Clothed and Totally Sober)
- **Naked Risk-Taking:** How to Always Win, Regardless of the Score
- **The Naked Roommate:** And Everything Else You Might Run Into in College
- **The Naked Roommate For Parents Only:** Everything Your Son or Daughter Will Run Into in College

For more information on Harlan's events, please visit him at www.DadsExpectingToo.com or www.HelpMeHarlan .com

INDEX

baby
    bonding with, 96–98, 380, 399, 400, 406, 415–417, 434–435
    caring for, 415–467. *See also* breastfeeding; safety
    development, 75–94
Baby Bargains (Fields), 264, 271, 272, 282–283, 284
babymoons, 225–229
baby-proofing services, 278–279
bedding, 265, 268, 423–424
bed rest, 62–64, 67, 68, 69, 125–126, 132, 145, 176
belly
    hanging out with, 87, 91, 243, 298–302
    button, baby's, 389
    button, pregnancy, 88, 152, 300
    touching, 129
birth
    announcing, 398, 406
    canal, 93, 94, 374–375, 377, 378–380, 387–388
    classes, 327–333, 335–336, 471
    coaches. *See* doulas; midwives
    defects. *See* prenatal testing
    facts and stats, 325
    locations, 14, 15, 18–22, 25, 470

    watching, 378–379, 386, 390–393
birth plans
    advocate, role of, 130, 333–334, 355, 356, 357–359, 380, 385, 405
    afterbirth, 381
    aftercare, 333, 380, 400, 405
    caregivers and, 15, 16, 17, 49, 323–327, 356, 357–359, 397, 400, 405
    cord blood banking, 340–344
    C-sections, 326–327, 385, 400
    hospital visitors, 339
    overview, 19, 323–327
    pain management, 348–355
    videotaping, 395–396, 397
birthing
    centers, 14, 19–20, 25, 470
    phase, 377–380
birthing vagina versus sex vagina, 43, 44, 46, 247, 391–392, 463
birthstones, 240
bisphenol A (BPA), 439
bladder control, loss of, 173, 174, 175, 245–246
bladder infection, 66–67
bonding, 96–98, 380, 399, 400, 406, 415–417, 434–435

partner, role of, 16, 113, 130, 331–336, 376, 377, 378, 379

stages of, 329, 375–382

See also contractions; delivery

lactation consultants, 27, 432–433, 436, 437, 471

Lamaze, 328, 335–336, 400, 471

lanugo, 85, 92

LATCH system, 281–282, 284

layettes, 262

leave

Family and Medical Leave Act (FMLA), 321

maternity, 23, 320–321

paternity, 316, 319–321, 472

leg cramps, 152, 156, 186

letdown, 434

linea nigra, 300

lingerie, 104, 236

listening to her belly, 300

Lullaby (Roberts), 445

M

magnets, 277

massages, 229–232, 243, 328

mastitis, 70

masturbation, 246, 258–260

maternal serum marker screening tests, 59–60

MaterniT21 testing, 58

Mayo Clinic Guide to a Health Pregnancy, 76, 114

meat, 33, 35–36

meconium, 94

MEDICAID, 29

medical resources, 114–115, 180, 470–472, 473–474

medical tests

newborn, 57, 400–404, 405, 474

prenatal, 23, 25, 49, 53, 55–61, 63, 92, 473–474

See also ultrasound

medicines, over-the-counter, 36

mental health, 168–169, 214–219

See also Depression

metabolic screening, 404

me-too complaining, 104, 134–136

midwives, 13–14, 15–17, 20, 25, 470

certified nurse-midwives, 16, 20

direct-entry midwives, 16, 20

registered nurse midwives, 16, 20

mind of pregnant woman, 189–219

mirror, use of, 378, 392–393

miscarriages, 9, 10, 58, 59, 61, 63, 70–74, 473

relationship changes, 71–72,
    101–102, 109, 110, 111,
    139–142, 419
rudeness, 128–129

S

safety
    bottles, 439
    car seats, 265, 282, 283,
        284–285, 471
    cribs, 265, 266, 277,
        279–280, 423, 424
    food, 32–33, 34, 35–36,
        129–130, 242, 472
    furniture assembly, 263–264,
        265, 275–277
    home hazards, 277–279
    infant CPR, 328, 329, 330,
        382, 471
    of prenatal tests, 58, 59, 61,
        63
    sex, 113–114, 246–248, 374
    SIDS, 423, 425
    sleep environment, 279–280,
        423–424, 427
    ultrasounds, 308
screening tests, 57–61, 404,
    474
seat belts, 228
selfishness, 106, 110
sex, 245–260
    after birth of baby, 46, 392,
        419, 461–463, 465

birthing vagina versus sex
    vagina, 43, 44, 46, 247,
        391–392, 463
guide to, 248–255
increasing chances of, 182,
    183, 222, 223, 230,
    231, 242, 248–249,
    251–252
inducing labor, 360, 361–362
masturbation, 246, 258–260
oral, 245–246
rejection, 98–102, 255–257
safety, 113–114, 246–248, 374
sex of baby, finding out, 27,
    51, 52, 53, 287–292
sexually transmitted diseases
    (STDs), 402–403
sex week checkup, 462
shopping, 211, 212, 261–285,
    472–473, 474. *See also
    specific item*
shopping timeline, 126–127,
    276
shushing, 426
sickle-cell anemia, 56, 474
SIDS (Sudden Infant Death
    Syndrome), 423, 425
skin-to-skin contact, 333,
    399, 400
sleep
    deprivation baby, caring for,
        143, 415–416, 418, 422–
        427, 429, 436, 444–448

ABOUT THE AUTHOR

Harlan Cohen is the bestselling author of five books, a professional speaker, and one of the most widely read and respected male syndicated advice columnists in the country.

He is the author of the books *The Naked Roommate: And 107 Other Issues You Might Run Into in College* (Sourcebooks), *The Naked Roommate: For Parents Only!* (Sourcebooks), *The Naked Roommate's First Year Survival Workbook* (Sourcebooks), *Getting Naked: Five Steps to Finding The Love of Your Life (While Fully Clothed and Totally Sober)* (St. Martin's Press), *Dad's Expecting Too!* (Sourcebooks), and *Campus Life Exposed: Advice from the Inside* (Peterson's). Harlan's writing and advice have been featured in the *New York Times*, *Wall Street Journal Classroom Edition*, *Cosmopolitan*, *Seventeen*, *Psychology Today*, and hundreds of other newspapers and publications. King

Features Syndicate distributes Harlan's "Help Me, Harlan!" advice column worldwide. He has been a guest on hundreds of radio and television programs, including the *Today Show*. Harlan is a professional speaker who has visited over four hundred college campuses. He is an expert who addresses teen issues, college life, conflict resolution, parenting, pregnancy, dating, relationships, sex, no sex, rejection, risk-taking, leadership, women's issues, and a variety of other topics.

Harlan is the founder of the websites www.Naked Roommate.com, www.GettingNakedExperiment.com, www.NakedRoommateForParents.com, www.DadsExpecting Too.com, and www.HelpMeHarlan.com. He is the producer and singer/songwriter on his album *Fortunate Accidents*.

He lives in Chicago, Illinois, with his pregnant wife, two young children, and dog. In his spare time, he thinks about how little spare time he has (and then his spare time is over, leaving him thinking about how he squandered his spare time, eating up more spare time).

Hey, thanks for spending your time (spare or not) reading this book and this bio.